THE ART OF PHARMACOECONOMICS

A Guide to Getting Started

Dr. ROLA KAAKEH

Copyright © 2021 Rola Kaakeh. All Rights Reserved.

No portion of this book may be reproduced or distributed. The reuse, storage, distribution, recording, translation or reproduction (verbal, written, electronic or mechanical) of any part of this publication, features, content, name, logo, designs, any service marks, and all original content in any form (current methods or developed in the future) is strictly prohibited without prior written approval and consent of the author and publisher.

First Edition: 2021
ISBN 978-1-7368386-0-0 (paperback edition)

Published by: Salus Vitae Group LLC
https://www.salusvitaegroup.com

To request permission, submit via the website https://www.salusvitaegroup.com to the publisher, with subject "Attention: Permission"

Disclaimer
Information is constantly evolving in the healthcare space. A responsible effort was made to provide accurate information from reliable sources at the time of publication. Information provided in the book is done so in good faith; however, no liabilities for the information (such as errors or omission) exist. The author and publisher disclaim any responsibility and are not liable (makes no guarantees or warranties, expressed or implied) for the accuracy, completeness, availability, and quality of the information and content ('content' includes, but is not limited to, the writing, statistics, figures, tables, graphs, references, and any images) provided. The reader should seek additional resources and professionals when appropriate. The reader should make their own assessment and determination of how they will use the information provided. The author and publisher provide no guarantees of any specific outcome or consequence as a result of utilizing recommendations or information offered in this book. This is not meant to provide medical advice or replace any consultation or discussion with your healthcare provider. The information is intended to enhance your knowledge and supplement existing tools. Readers are advised to continuously check the latest updates, information, practices, and guidelines.

To my family,
I'm endlessly grateful and indebted to you for your encouragement, love, mentorship and inspiration.

To my colleagues, mentors, and thought-leaders,
thank you for all you have taught me over the years and your contributions to advancing healthcare and public health.

Preface	i

SECTION 1: DECISION-MAKING AND PHARMACOECONOMICS — 9

CHAPTER 1: INTRODUCTION — 11
- Scarcity and Allocation of Resources — 11
- Realities on the Ground versus Goals — 15
- Value — 21
- Decision-Making — 28
- Decision-Making Questionnaire — 34
- Up Next — 38

CHAPTER 2: A FOCUS ON OUTCOMES — 39
- Healthcare – Innovation – Outcomes (HIO) Triad — 39
- Outcomes Research — 41
- Efficacy or Effectiveness? — 45
- Using Evidence in Real-World Decision-Making — 47
- Up Next — 52

CHAPTER 3: PHARMACOECONOMICS — 53
- Basics of Health Economics — 53
- What is Pharmacoeconomics (PE)? — 53
- Significance & Rise of Pharmacoeconomics — 55
- Role of PE Analyses in Decision-Making — 56
- Issues with the Use of PE Analyses — 59
- How We Learn Pharmacoeconomics — 61
- Up Next — 61

CHAPTER 4: ECONOMICS ANALYSES — 63
- Overview of Economic Analyses — 63
- Cost-Minimization Analysis — 65
- Cost-Benefit Analysis — 67
- Cost-Effectiveness Analysis — 70
- Cost-Utility Analysis — 75
- Other Types: Cost of Illness — 78
- Other Types: Cost Consequence Analysis — 78
- Other Types: Budget Impact Analysis — 79
- Up Next — 79

SECTION 2: DESIGNING, CONDUCTING, AND EVALUATING PHARMACOECONOMICS ANALYSES — 81

CHAPTER 5: DESIGNING AND CURATING THE EXPERIENCE — 83

- Researchers are Designers — 83
- Lifecycle of a Pharmacoeconomics Analysis — 86
- Pharmacoeconomics Base — 88
- Domains of The Process — 97
- Elements of The Process — 99
- Up Next — 105

CHAPTER 6: BUILDING THE TEAM — 107

- Team Types — 108
- Team Archetypes — 111
- Characteristics of the Team Members — 117
- Recruiting Team Members — 121
- Team Assessments — 122
- Designing the Team Experience — 124
- Design Meetings — 125
- Up Next — 128

CHAPTER 7: THE PHARMACOECONOMICS CANVAS — 129

- Guidance on Pharmacoeconomics Analyses — 129
- Introduction to the Pharmacoeconomics Canvas — 131
- An Approach to Conduct and Evaluate PE Analyses — 133
- How to Use the Pharmacoeconomics Canvas — 134
- The Pharmacoeconomics Canvas — 137
- Frame 1: Define the Criteria — 139
- Frame 2: Frame the Methods then Conduct and/or Evaluate — 156
- Frame 3: Evaluate the Output — 186
- Up Next — 194

SECTION 3: PUTTING IT ALL TOGETHER — 195

- Brief Summary of the Book — 196
- Abbreviations — 198
- References — 201
- Index — 213

Preface

Why was the book written?

Professionals within the healthcare space provide numerous value-added products and services – such as life-saving procedures and medications. Nevertheless, many healthcare decisions are not made solely on demonstrated clinical outcomes but rather include cost, quality of life, and patient-preferences measures. How much are you willing to pay to save a life or extend life for a year? What should policymakers and society be willing to pay for an additional or incremental unit of health gain? If you feel apprehensive about answering these questions, you are not alone. Who would not feel strained with answering these questions or making such decisions? Many healthcare professionals are uncomfortable due to the "save a life mentality" they are trained to have and feel they must do what is required for maximal health gains.

We must not minimize the reality of limited, finite resources. Our heightened awareness of this forces us to be judicious with the use of our resources. Professionals must be intentional with value creation due to endlessly competing options available. There are various products and services constantly competing for and demanding our attention. A trade-off should be made.

As we continue to juggle the growing, fast-paced advancements in technology, innovation, and disruptions, it is essential to summarize and simplify the fundamentals of how we demonstrate and communicate value. Healthcare providers are often driven to achieve improved clinical outcomes due to their strong clinical background. However, many professionals lack the training to communicate better and articulate that value beyond being merely descriptive in nature or focusing on only one outcome. Numerous professionals still lack the skill sets needed to tell their value stories in a more targeted, meaningful way to decision-makers. It is expected of all professionals to learn new skills and foster innovative, transformative, unconventional thinking to add value and remain relevant in this face-paced environment.

We have seen a rise in outcomes research conducted over the past few decades. Outcomes research is a broad, complex, and holistic methodological discipline that aims to provide effectiveness data about the benefits, results, and real-world impact of interventions in

Preface

practice. It has become a necessity in the healthcare sector – both from a system and personnel standpoint – to acquire the skills to conduct and evaluate this research. There is a call to demonstrate the value of the products and services provided.

Traditional training of outcomes research remains limited and has failed to reach everyone. These trainings have included instructions in the classroom setting, textbooks, additional graduate-level degrees, such as masters or doctorates, and post-graduate training, such as fellowships. We also see a greater emphasis on outcomes research and pharmacoeconomics within the healthcare professional school curriculum (e.g., pharmacy schools). However, there continues to be a limited number of professionals with expertise and training in this field.

Historically, the ideas and methods of the discipline are presented the same way – in the form of textbooks that read similarly and contain the same information. Several technical books go through the methodology of the science of pharmacoeconomics and outcomes research in detail. The intensely technical literature, while extremely valuable, acts as a barrier for many health professionals to create, understand, and use the information generated by pharmacoeconomic analyses. Many are apprehensive even about getting started.

While many resources for conducting and evaluating pharmacoeconomic analyses exist, they still lack a clear, holistic, simple bird's eye view approach to summarizing the common elements involved in the discipline's foundation of research-creation, evaluation, and communication. I could not find any book that spoke to the broad, simple macro-level of the varied elements that go into pharmacoeconomics research and practice, particularly how you get started, and the personnel required. Such an approach was something I looked for personally before embarking on my fellowship. We must approach this topic in a new way to allow for greater use of the information and involvement of healthcare professionals in this field. There is a need to see the "world of pharmacoeconomics" in all of its facets. To understand what it would take to perform and evaluate these types of analyses (from the content to the teams and ultimately to communicating the information). Efforts must be made to cultivate the need to understand the art of pharmacoeconomics.

The goal of the book

The goal is to simplify a complex discipline to break down the skills gaps and competency barriers faced by healthcare professionals. It serves as an easy-to-read guide to the key elements that go into the process of conducting and evaluating pharmacoeconomic analyses and provides the reader with the framework and tools needed. It will help the reader familiarize themselves with the various components and elements of pharmacoeconomics. It will simplify the process and provide you with the tools (including the PE lifecycle, domains, and canvas) to get started – which you can use on your path to assess the outcomes and value of interventions.

This book aims to build the capacity and unlock potential for all health professionals working to achieve better outcomes and greater value. It provides a starting point for individuals looking to grow their competencies and skills in health outcomes research, focusing on pharmacoeconomics. Now, more than ever, professionals must be purposeful with how they create, evaluate, and communicate outcomes and value. The hope is to empower and make it easier for more healthcare professionals to perform, evaluate, and incorporate pharmacoeconomic analyses into their practice and decision-making.

The objective of the book is that you see the world of healthcare decision-making a little differently and cultivate a growing community around the need for this topic. This book speaks to the art, and not just the technical features, of the discipline.

I believe this discipline is an art form, and you are a designer or artist. Learning the art of pharmacoeconomics in the manner addressed in the book will help tell stories of impact through a more objective and evidence-based approach. The book contents may serve as a foundation for sharing, deploying, learning, motivating, and discussing this field's components.

Who should read this book?

This book is designed for students, residents, healthcare and public health professionals, and decision-makers. Everyone, regardless of prior expertise or background in pharmacoeconomics and outcomes research, would benefit from learning the skills and fundamentals taught in this book.

Preface

These skills apply to individuals practicing in all settings and specialties. It is great for organizations looking to train their professionals on the path to getting started to create, demonstrate, evaluate, and communicate outcomes and value. It is written in such a way that any individual may easily understand the fundamentals with no in-depth knowledge or expertise in this field. No matter what stage you are in your career, you must acquire these skills for the work you do to continue to be relevant and sustainable in the present and future.

The elements outlined in the book are meant for the visionaries in healthcare and those who are "disrupting" the way we strive to achieve better health outcomes. These include individuals:

- Looking for novel ways to improve outcomes, access, quality, and reduce costs.
- Envisioning innovative solutions but are looking to broaden their scope and skills to track, demonstrate, and communicate the value of the products and interventions.
- Looking to answer questions such as, "Are our decisions evidence-based?"

These individuals recognize that healthcare cannot move forward without demonstrating the value and sustainability of our interventions. They understand that it is crucial that we carefully design our interventions and make more efficient use of current and future resources.

Innovators look to transform and improve their institutions and communities and recognize they should commit to building their skills set and focus on professional development. There is an endless, noteworthy need to cultivate talent and become scientifically creative within healthcare. As healthcare professionals reinvent themselves, create products, and start new practices or services, they need to grow and continuously acquire new skills. Professionals must move up in their abilities and build the analytical and technical expertise to demonstrate outcomes and, ultimately, value. The ability to conduct pharmacoeconomics and outcomes research and work with professionals from various backgrounds will increase our reach as healthcare professionals to continue creating and demonstrating outcomes and value.

Recognizing that not all healthcare professionals will conduct pharmacoeconomic analyses, many, however, will be required to read and evaluate this type of research. It is vital to become familiar with the terminology, processes, and methods to acquire the knowledge to assess and practically apply the concepts into a professional's thought process.

Overall, this book is for self-directed lifelong learners who are looking to:
- Broaden their scope of skills and build a holistic skill set to better inform decisions, tackle the challenges facing healthcare, and create transformational improvements.
- Utilize objective methods to inform healthcare decisions.
- Discover what other skills are continuously needed among healthcare professionals.

If you make any decisions in healthcare, then this book is for you. Anyone who ultimately has the power to make any decision in healthcare needs to equip themselves with the skills to conduct or, at the very least, evaluate outcomes research – of which pharmacoeconomics is a type. This book for every healthcare professional who wants to show up, innovate, chart their course, and contribute to value-added, sustainable interventions for their patients, institutions, and communities.

How to use this book

Readers can use the contents of the book, both in the classroom and in practice, to
- Learn the discipline of pharmacoeconomics and outcomes research
- Conduct and evaluate pharmacoeconomics studies
- Supplement existing pharmacoeconomics resources

As you go through the book, you will begin to learn about key concepts and understand pharmacoeconomics as a craft, with all of its components pieced together. The chapters highlight the elements and skills that students, practitioners, administrators, and institutions need to equip themselves when conducting and evaluating pharmacoeconomic analyses. The reader should use this book as a roadmap to create an "outcomes and value state of mind." Empty pages are available for note-taking at the end of the book. Professionals will learn how to leverage data to articulate the outcomes and value of a product and intervention.

This book is not meant to replace the technical methods-based books or articles – as it cannot replace these resources. It is intended to complement existing resources designed to develop further and train future researchers in this field. Pharmacoeconomics is a science, and more information and explanations are needed to conduct this research appropriately.

Scope of the book

The *Art of Pharmacoeconomics* is the first of its kind that takes a macro-level approach to the methodology, skills, and personnel needed to perform and evaluate pharmacoeconomic research. These analyses can be very time-consuming, complex, and labor-intensive. It provides the reader with a high-level, bird's eye view of the starting concepts and elements of pharmacoeconomics needed to perform and evaluate this type of work. It uses a holistic approach to simplify the complexity, making it straightforward enough to get started and integrate it into a busy practitioner's thought process and practice. It will provide you an essential beginner's fundamental understanding of the principles to articulate, work on, evaluate studies, and use these tools and information in practice and decision-making when needed. This abridged method will allow the reader to quickly learn fundamental concepts and apply them in practice when needed.

This book complements the recommendations made by existing resources and incorporates several other key elements, processes, and methods associated with pharmacoeconomics. This book uses a simplified approach to motivate more professionals to take on and learn about this discipline.

Summary of the book

The book is organized into three sections.

- **Section 1: Decision-Making and Pharmacoeconomics** - serves as a background and introduces the concept of healthcare resource allocation, value, decision-making, outcomes research, and pharmacoeconomics analyses.
- **Section 2: Designing, Conducting, and Evaluating Pharmacoeconomics Analyses** - goes through the process of designing, conducting, and evaluating pharmacoeconomics analyses. It also features information on how to go about building a team, whom you should consider working/or partnering with, and why. The Lifecycle of Pharmacoeconomics, Pharmacoeconomics Base, Domains and Elements of The Process, and the Pharmacoeconomics Canvas are introduced and summarized in this section.
- **Section 3: Putting it All Together** - provides information on abbreviations, references, index, and empty pages for notes.

The book is written in "active writing" and colloquial language to reflect on how one would teach this subject in real-life and practice. Several self-reflection questions will be built-in throughout the book, allowing the reader to evaluate current activities and project them onto future goals. Take a moment – as you get to them throughout the book – to answer the items in the various chapters and sections.

What is not within the scope of the book

This book is an introduction to the fundamentals and should be used as a resource or reference book. It is meant to serve as a roadmap – "state of mind" – and not a "rule book" and is not intended to be prescriptive. The book is meant to be a beginner's guide to getting started and is <u>not</u> a complete, all-inclusive reference on the discipline of pharmacoeconomics or outcomes research. It is not a textbook but rather more a "how-to" guidebook that you can use for your self-development of this discipline.

Many of the concepts and methods highlighted in this book are foundational concepts and may require additional resources to grasp fully. For example, many statistical tests and specific methodological approaches are mentioned but are not covered in detail in the book. You will need to resort to additional resources for information on methods. Professionals are encouraged to add it to their resources as they construct their unique toolkits to acquire the skills they need. When publishing this type of research in peer-reviewed journals, I recommend that the reader consult the journal to see the format, methodology criteria, and reporting requirements and not just rely on this book's content. Make it a habit to continuously check the most current best practices in the world of pharmacoeconomics and outcomes research. I encourage you to seek out resources beyond this book frequently.
Now, let's get started!

SECTION 1: DECISION-MAKING AND PHARMACOECONOMICS

CHAPTER 1: INTRODUCTION

Scarcity and Allocation of Resources

We must not minimize the reality of limited, finite resources. Our heightened awareness of resource scarcity forces us to be judicious with their use. There are various products and services constantly competing for and demanding our attention. A trade-off should be made. We all make allocation decisions – decisions on what, how, and to whom we spend our time and resources. One may even contemplate how much they are willing to pay to solve an issue. We think of the value or the output of our options. We have to choose among these options and ultimately make a decision. We need to help prioritize efforts and utilization of resources to maximize health outcomes. The concepts and need to appropriately distribute resources efficiently translate across all disciplines, making it so essential.

The allocation of resources requires discipline. On both an individual and systemic level, one should be disciplined in allocating resources to strategically optimize their contribution to both the institution's business and the patients' health. When equipped with better information, we can more efficiently assign resources. For something to be sustainable, the value should be demonstrated; otherwise, resources may not be re-allocated to (continue) the intervention we perceive to be beneficial. Several facets go into systematically assessing the value of products and services.

We make decisions every day, and as leaders, we often make decisions that determine the future of ideas, products, services, jobs, and our professions or discipline as a whole. We create plans to respond to our patients' current and future needs, disciplines, settings, and communities.

An overarching goal should be to provide more objective, evidence-based decision-making in healthcare. To do this effectively, we need to understand our environments and how we are making decisions.

Chapter 1: Introduction

How much are you willing to pay to save a life or extend life for a year? What should policymakers and society be willing to pay for an additional or incremental unit of health gain? If you feel apprehensive about answering these questions, you are not alone. Who would not feel strained with answering these questions or making such decisions? Many healthcare professionals are uncomfortable due to the "save a life mentality" they are trained to have and feel they must do what is required for maximal health gains.

What if you are answering these questions as the payer or a patient? Would your answers change? A **critical** question to answer here is, who bears the cost? The individual or institution that often bears the cost drives many of the allocation decisions. They ultimately determine how much and to what they will assign resources. There is no societal consensus about how much money to spend on any particular item.

Given the responsibility of clinicians and administrators to be judicious with their resources, there is a need to make sure they are efficiently used and understand and evaluate the basis for their decision.[1-9] The responsibility to ensure proper use of resources is not limited to specific healthcare professionals. It is the shared responsibility of all stakeholders – e.g., healthcare providers, professionals, payers, and society as a whole.

Healthcare is falling behind meeting public expectations and values. There is a need to shift from a system centered on the volume of consumption to a focus on products and services that provide value and improve health. There is a call to action to change from volume-based thinking (or doing more, increasing the quantity or use of more products and services) to a value mindset.[7,10-20] We see more conversations around value-based vs. volume-based decision-making in healthcare.

Value looks at what you are paying for and not just what you are paying.[20] More on this topic later in this chapter. We are obliged to enhance our healthcare systems in ways that add value.

There is never a "blank check" in healthcare, so how do we objectively decide where to allocate our resources? In environments where resources are limited, we care to minimize waste and optimize expenses and time to high-value products or services. The perfect scenario would be to only invest in high-value items, resulting in high returns and costs less than others. Such circumstances do not exist for every decision situation experienced. Decision-making is often not as straightforward.

Develop a growth-oriented strategy by focusing on value.

There is an art to balancing value and costs or expenses. We should identify what approaches we are using to create a system to prioritize and de-prioritize products and services. Start getting into a mindset of prioritizing products and services of greater value and de-prioritizing those of less value.[7,13,21]

Examples of low-value care, highlighted by the Task Force on Low-Value Care, include using expensive brand name medications (when an identical active ingredient generic are available), prostate-specific antigen screening in men 75 years of age and older, population-based vitamin D screening, and diagnostic testing before low-risk surgery for low-risk patients.[14-17] We are seeing a high volume of low-value care, which leads to a significant waste of resources, increases in delays and patient harms, and has financial implications on health systems, payers, and patients.[14,15]

According to the Center for Value-Based Insurance Design, high-value services are those with improved clinical outcomes, efficiency, and robust evidence base.[22] Examples provided include hemoglobin A1c tests, blood pressure monitors, high-value prescription drugs, pulmonary rehabilitation, diabetic foot exams, and lower cost-sharing.[17,23,24]

The financial burden that healthcare places, the greater availability and accessibility of health information, and the increased focus on providing patient-centered care have allowed patients to take more autonomy and ownership for decision-making.[7,13,25,26]

By building a value-based approach to decision making, individuals can make better allocation decisions with the lens of what adds value.

Healthcare decisions are made quickly and within specific **time frames**. Timing is everything, and even a previously functioning process may only work temporarily. With new information, we have the opportunity to self-evaluate, pivot, and innovate to improve outcomes. Why? Because there is a high level of urgency – lives are at stake, and lives matter.[27] One should recognize the urgency associated with allocation and decision-making in general within these settings. Consider using a deliberative, structured process to assist with measuring and communicating value to make objective decisions. Such a method allows for additional resources to be directed towards resources that have a higher value. Be able to answer how you are repositioning yourself and your institution to meet your patients' needs and the growing demands of an ever-changing healthcare landscape.

Human Resources

Not only do we use allocation principles for budgets and investments in products and services, but also in the hiring, positioning, and evaluation of healthcare personnel. Investing in the innovation of workforce development is critical to achieving better health outcomes.

Train and build the competencies of professionals to begin to shift to value-centric thinking.

Training decision-makers and professionals in the proficiencies of objective, deliberative value analysis is an investment for the future – as this allows them to translate the results into practice to reduce wasteful spending and improve the quality of care.[7,28] Therefore, anyone who ultimately has the power to make any decision in healthcare needs to equip themselves with the skills to conduct or, at the very least, evaluate outcomes research (OR). More on Outcomes Research can be found in Chapter 2.

Realities on the Ground versus Goals

Healthcare is complex and ever-changing. Healthcare consumes a significant amount of countrywide spending. Overall, the United States (US) spent an estimated $3.6 trillion on healthcare in 2018, spending significantly more than any other country.[29-35] Medications are a large share of health budgets.[13,25] The US total prescription spending is estimated to have reached $476 billion in 2018 – this is comparable to the full economies of some developed countries.[30,36,37] However, the amount we spend is not directly correlated with the quality of care or better health outcomes.

Healthcare systems struggle with vulnerable and fragmented environments – ones that consist of several operational and systemic flaws. We often juggle between what is currently happening on the ground and our goals.

Realities on the ground = what you currently have
Our realities reflect what is on the ground – which can vary based on institution.

Goals = what you would like to achieve
These goals encompass the views and perspectives of all stakeholders. We should create a system that rewards achieving the goals. The goals drive and propel us.

The goal of many is to design cost-conscious interventions that add value.

To achieve our goals, one should have a comprehensive multi-level strategy that utilizes various tools to build and foster the ideal environment to achieve these objectives. We need to work to ensure patients are getting better in the highest quality, efficient, cost-effective, and clinically appropriate manner possible. We understand the value that results from providing healthcare to overall health.

The path to improvement uses metrics that must be constantly tested and evaluated. We collect information, analyze it, and then communicate this information to our teams. We develop tools, report cards, protocols, best practices, and action plans tailored to our target outcomes. The purpose is to identify weaknesses in our systems, draw out organizational structures and connections, identify areas where potential or actual errors occur, identify gaps in communication, and map out new methods of communication.[27]

Chapter 1: Introduction

Examine your current realities and your future goals.

Start by answering the following questions:
- Where is the healthcare sector going?
- What are the problems or challenges faced in healthcare?
- What are your goals? Determine what is relevant to your environment.
- What measures are appropriate for your situation?
- What are the drivers?
- What are the industry needs?
- How are we solving the issues identified?
- Are we utilizing multi-factorial and multi-level strategies?
- What skill sets are you lacking?
- Are we building holistic skill sets (skills of today and the future)?
- What are we doing to train professionals?
- How are and will we interact with technology and data?

We need to understand and outline an organization's current needs, goals, and priorities. Many institutions' ultimate goal is to design our systems to improve efficiency, convenience, health outcomes, quality, access, satisfaction, experience, add value, and cut costs.

Briefly outlined below are a few current realities across seven healthcare target categories – items that are often evaluated within healthcare. These are then compared with the broad goals of many healthcare professionals and institutions. There are complexities and barriers to achieving the desired goals in these categories. Consider reviewing each category at your institution and add to or remove them as needed. Summarize what is being done now and the impact on your outcomes of interest. What skills are necessary to fulfill future needs? What are you doing now to address any gaps? Where can you grow or adapt to meet your objectives and goals? You will also need to evaluate the skills set available at your institution to make the goals a reality.

Seven Healthcare Target Categories

Category 1: Health Outcomes

Realities

- Desired health outcomes may not always be met due to several systemic or individual barriers.

Goals

- Improve and reach desired or target patient health outcomes.
- Improve survival and quality of life (QOL).

Category 2: Efficiency

Realities

- Complex and fragmented systems. Fragmentation leads to uncertain ownership of the responsibility to ensure the appropriate use of resources overall. Consider asking: is the system fragmented or straightforward enough to be controlled?
- Multiple payers and systems with a mix of public and private payers (pluralistic).

Goals

- Streamline processes. Improve efficiency with the current and expansion of products and services. Develop infrastructure when and where required.
- Utilize technology and innovative practices to track real-world data and use it to assist with evidence-based decision-making.

Category 3: Quality

Realities

- Low quality or questionable quality is present. Quality is exceptionally variable across healthcare settings. Determine what and where you are comfortable with paying more to achieve higher quality.

Goals

- High quality – to achieve and maintain high-quality products and services. Better quality leads to better experiences and outcomes.
- Desire to keep quality high and costs low. We do not want to decrease quality when we implement cost-containment strategies. At the very least, we must be cognizant of how quality changes when we incorporate interventions.

Chapter 1: Introduction

Category 4: Cost

Realities

- High costs of products and services. High healthcare expenditures overall, which continue to rise.
- Costs linked to innovation – e.g., high costs associated with new technologies or new medications. The effects of increases in technology on cost are apparent. Additional spending will continue as innovation increases.
- Budget challenges and constraints – limited budgets or restrictive budgets. One can technically cut costs by deciding not to fund something, leading to the debate between underutilization and cost containment strategies. However, the consequences of doing this on health should not be overlooked.

Goals

- Lower costs. Identify cost containment strategies to help manage rising costs. Cost avoidance strategies can come in many forms, including decreasing readmissions, costs of complications, and sequence of events.
- Find ways to best utilize the costly innovation created and adopted. Keep costs down while allowing for innovation and advancement in technology.
- Limited budgets will always remain – therefore, one should continuously utilize strategies to manage budget challenges efficiently.
- Allocate those expenditures to resources that add value. With rising costs and restrictive budgets, we need to be smarter in using our limited resources.
- The focus of all individuals, institutions, and systems is to reduce healthcare costs; therefore, economic data must be incorporated into the assessment of value and decision-making, along with the other clinical and safety endpoints.

Category 5: Equity

Realities

- Access to and coverage for all healthcare products and services for all individuals remains limited.
- Disparities in access and health outcomes exist.

Goals

- Increase access to healthcare products and services.
- Achieve equitable access to healthcare products and services.

Category 6: Satisfaction and Experience

Realities
- Variable, questionable, uneven satisfaction of products and services provided.
- Not a consistent priority across healthcare settings.
- There is a need to manage both provider and patient preferences.
- The more that innovation becomes individualized, the more it costs.

Goals
- Achieve greater satisfaction and better experiences within the healthcare system.
- Improve the patient and healthcare professional experience.
- Provide more individualized care, with the patient as an integral part of the decision-making process. The future will be more personalized, thus recognizing what will work for specific patients (and providers) is essential.

Category 7: Value

Realities
- Uncertain value overall – or at least, value is not always explicitly communicated.
- Continuous debate over the benefits and impact of volume-based reimbursement system vs. value-based reimbursement systems.

Goals
- Create, demonstrate, and communicate the value of the products and services within healthcare.
- Consider incorporating value-based strategies or methods.
- Increase value-added products and services to enhance value to patients, practices, institutions, and other stakeholders.

Chapter 1: Introduction

We face numerous challenges – challenges to which we should rise. Our goal should be to achieve better health and not just provide better healthcare.

The World Health Organization (WHO) defined human health in a broader sense in its 1948 constitution as "a state of complete physical, mental and social well-being and not merely the absence of disease or infirmity."[38] Merely having access to healthcare products and services is not a guarantee for improved health. We know there is more to an individual's health than the healthcare we provide them. This reality poses a challenge for all of us, as we must all step up and address the numerous social determinants of health that are negatively impacting our well-being. There are spillover effects of each intervention we make in healthcare to another sector.[39] Thus, we should also focus on multiple industries and evaluate how the interventions could potentially work in these sectors. It is also essential to assess the ripple effects of each decision and intervention on the whole system – to see if it enables or hinders access and quality of care and at what cost. We have to identify the appropriate strategies to simultaneously address multiple issues and realities, both locally and globally.

Value

Value has been defined by health economists "as what individuals (or others acting on their behalf) would be willing to pay to acquire more health care or other goods or services."[40,41] If you take a basic definition that looks at value as the result of evaluating outcomes or benefits over costs, you will notice that the higher the benefits and lower the costs, the greater the value.[1,21,41]

When you see healthcare as an investment rather than an expense, you start asking the value question. Priority should be given to allocating and positioning your resources to the people and items that demonstrate the most value for your institutions and those you serve.

As we begin to juggle the growing, fast-paced advancements in technology, innovation, and disruptions, it is essential to summarize and simplify the fundamentals of how we demonstrate and communicate value. Professionals have a duty to be intentional with value creation. Incentivizing value is crucial to building interventions that create a measurable and lasting impact. Do not just look for new ways to cut costs but look for new ways to distribute resources to items that add value – however you may define value. We must develop the competencies and skills needed to plan for the present and future needs effectively.

The WHO updated its Essential Medicines List in 2019 "to guide decisions about which medicines represent the best value for money, based on evidence and health impact," – said WHO Director-General Dr. Tedros Adhanom Ghebreyesus.[54] This list includes 460 essential products and is used by more than 150 countries to assist with prioritizing products to address public health conditions.[54]

Value is multidimensional and highly dependent on the decision context and the perspective of the individual or group defining it. It varies significantly among different stakeholders.[2,27,41-50] Value embodies a broad collection of factors and experiences relevant to and utilized by individuals, institutions, and society. Those who pay for and receive a product or service are concerned with the value they extract from them. What does the "person" care about? We answer this to assess if this provides them that value. For example, payers and health systems are usually interested in cost reduction.

Chapter 1: Introduction

Individuals and populations as a whole can value each item very differently. People differ in preferences, their willingness to pay, and what they are willing to trade.[26,41] There is an opportunity cost associated with decisions we make – meaning, we forgo a benefit obtained from the alternative choice to choose this one.[2,40,42,52,53]

We know that there is heterogeneity (i.e., diversity) and individual-level variations within these populations.[26,41,42,51] The data collected or available in the literature often reflect population averages; however, when you start to break these populations down into subgroups, you see individual-level variations.

Variation in individual value exists due to the numerous "elements of value" each "person" (individuals or organizations) places – or items they value or are important to them – and the differences in what they are willing to trade for each element. For example, what an individual is willing to trade to live shorter with a better QOL or more years with poorer QOL.[41]

Examples of "elements of value" identified in the literature include:[20,21,40,42,49]
- Improved clinical outcomes, such as survival, life-years gained
- Reduced severity of the disease and burden of disease
- Improved QOL
- Cost savings within and outside of health systems
- Improved productivity
- Equity
- Value of knowing, the value of hope, and "peace of mind"
- Insurance

Additional research is needed to understand how to measure many of these elements.[42]

Nevertheless, whoever ultimately pays needs to assess the value of those choices and make a decision. Insurance companies, hospitals, and clinicians act on behalf of patients to choose products that they believe are the best value for the money. Shared decision-making gives voice to the patient's perspective. Patients care about clinical outcomes but also care about other items such as quality of life, the burden of the disease, and worker productivity.[20,21] Regardless of the decision-maker's perspective, be sure the elements that are important to patients are accounted for within the decision-making process.

Differences with Value

The topic of value is often debated due to its heterogeneity of definitions, measurements, and decision recommendations. This has resulted in inconsistencies across frameworks and methods. Everyone is capturing value differently because everyone defines it differently. When you have varied definitions of value, then your proposed solutions may also look inconsistent. Therefore, the importance we place on a product or service can dramatically vary by individuals.[26,41,42,52] Assess individual value goals for products and services and compare them with how they align with organizational goals.

The issue or difficulty with setting one number or measure for value is that you limit individual variations in preferences by doing so.[41] Preferences influence what people value and drive decision-making.

Assess whether "value" is part of the decision equation. As a leader and decision-maker, have you defined what value means to you? Have you created a list of items that you value? Each institution and individual should be able to speak to the items that are important to them. By defining and mapping out value, you focus on improving and achieving better outcomes. You should have a process to evaluate value. In the process, you may notice untapped opportunities that add value.

The Need to Demonstrate Value

Several reasons exist for why the value of healthcare services should be demonstrated:
- Changes to the provision of healthcare. This includes changes to healthcare laws and policies, as well as the expanding role of providers. We should consistently track and evaluate the impact of these changes on patient outcomes.
- Addition of new products and replacement of the old. The advances in healthcare are leading to more new products and replacing the old.
- Resource limitations and prioritization. We are regularly asked to justify the investment and sustainability of products, professional programs, and other value-added services due to limited resources.

There is an ongoing need to find new ways to add value and further understand how we perceive and measure value and impact. The goal of demonstrating the value of a product or service is to help inform decision-making.[1]

Chapter 1: Introduction

Decision-makers are often asked to decide if a new intervention's higher costs are worth the added benefits. It would help if you looked beyond what you are willing to pay and the expense of acquiring a product or starting a service. Professionals often focus so much on "what is being done?" without asking, "what is adding value?" It is critical to add the value question to your operations.

There is a need to think of and continuously ask yourself:
- Are you getting value for your money? This question is critical when resources are low. As you continue spending money, consider answering the question: are the outcomes improving, staying the same, or getting worse?
- What is the value proposition? What value is this product, service, or intervention providing?
- To whom is the benefit going? You care about identifying value to whom – what does that "person" care about in the end?
- Who is paying, and who is getting the benefit? They may be the same person, but often they are not.
- What happens when the majority of the costs are now, but benefits are later? When do you see the benefits? What does that mean for the person paying (e.g., insurance companies)? Keep in mind; you may not be the one benefiting – perspective matters.
- How can we measure the value of our money now and in the long-term?
- How can you continue to grow, streamline, and add value?

A **"Value Process"** consists of three domains: creating, demonstrating, and communicating value.
1. **Creating** interventions such as products, programs, and services that add value.
2. **Demonstrating** the value through the implementation and evaluation of the interventions. Tools, such as cost-effectiveness analysis (CEA), are used to measure value.[9,19,41]
3. **Communicating** the value by first defining the audience or perspective, summarizing results, and making a recommendation to inform decision-making.

The time you spend performing each of these domains depends on the person, institution, need, or question at hand.

Several methods are used to demonstrate the value of services and interventions. The first step in measuring impact is identifying which "world" you are trying to impact to understand the perspective from which to tailor the perceived value metrics. That is, you are evaluating or determining the value to whom? And how does that person or group define value? A world can be your world (yourself), the world of a specific community you serve, or the global community as a whole. It would help if you outlined the gains or outcomes you hope to achieve based on this world's identified needs. Examples of product and service gains include the capacity to lower cost, improve access, improve efficiency, deliver greater health benefits, and provide higher quality care. You can create the operational pathways necessary to achieve a more significant impact when you have identified where the value lies.[50]

Wiser decisions around how we allocate our resources are warranted. There is an art to balancing value and cost expenditures. Ultimately the decision made should be seen as an investment; therefore, invest in what yields immense benefits.

Value Assessment Frameworks

With the desire by many within healthcare to become a more value-based system (rather than the current volume-based system), tools have emerged to assist with evaluating value.[7,10-20,55] "Value Frameworks" have appeared more frequently in the last few years in the United States as a tool to help with determining value.[7,21,26,48,55,56] Value assessment frameworks are one of these tools designed to help support the complex decision-making processes in healthcare.[20,40,48,55] They can be used by patients, providers, and payers and can focus on patient-level and plan-level decision-making. The framework assists payers in supporting coverage, pricing reimbursement decisions, designing clinical pathways, and shared decision-making process.[20,42,55,57]

We have shifted to more patient-centered care and increased shared decision-making, leading to the availability of patient-oriented value frameworks. Patient-oriented value frameworks have emerged to inform patients regarding costs and benefits, thereby recognizing patient preferences play a role in decision-making.[42] With the readily available information sources, patients are more informed, and we see them advocate for shared-decision-making (or clinician-patient level decision-making).[8,20] Choosing a therapy or course of action is often a shared decision. The process to consider patient preferences must be included in value frameworks.

Chapter 1: Introduction

The frameworks are diverse in their perspectives, definition of value, target decision-makers, measures included, analytical techniques, and decision thresholds.[21,40-42,55] Much of the criticism regarding these value assessment frameworks are rooted in that a different organization creates each value assessment.[19,40,42,45,52,55] The various frameworks available were developed to relay how the authors and organizations define and measure value. Each of these organizations have varying perspectives and goals. The purpose and use of the framework can depend on the perspective. Some agencies publish recommendations to assist in clinician-patient shared decision-making and construct standard of care guidelines and pathways that provide the most value.[40,41,45,55,56,58] While others target payers making health plans and reimbursement decisions (e.g., what drugs to cover).[40,41,45,55]

Perspective matters, as there are variations in priorities, missions, services, interventions, and processes based on the perspectives. Differences in perspectives, value definitions, decision criteria result in differences in decisions made.[40,42,52,55] The perspective can determine the decision threshold, how much budget is available, and how it is used. Opportunities to improve and update them continue by all stakeholders involved in creating and using these frameworks. Further understanding of the diversity of these tools assists in critiquing the assessment for use. When you define value differently, your measures vary, and the decisions that result from the variations in these two differ.

Be critical of any value assessment you may come across. Evaluate each framework to identify the perspective, audience, value definition, methods and metrics, assumptions, source of data, decision context, and decision criteria (how they decide) before incorporating the results. The source and process from which each of these elements was derived need to be transparent.[40,42,45,55]

It would be best to note how each organization framework defines and measures the various elements to decide. Ask yourself, what is impacting the results? Assumptions are made when all the evidence is not there; therefore, be sure to evaluate when and how assumptions are made critically. Recognize when these frameworks either oversimplify or make extreme assumptions, as some make assumptions with a lack of transparency on the quality or source of the data.[40]

Value

IMPORTANT:
No single assessment, checklist, or guidelines will work for every decision question.

Decision-Making

We are always faced with choices and asked to select based on what we are trying to achieve – such as improved health outcomes, higher profits, or better quality of care. With further progress and innovation, we will continue to experience multiple competing choices and questions. We will need to decide if and where to invest. We are faced with difficult questions every day – like, what should policymakers and society be willing to pay for an additional or incremental unit of health gain?

How do we make decisions? The decision-making process is multidimensional. Many healthcare professionals use instinct and clinical judgment to make decisions based on their education and experiences.[13,59] It is essential to move beyond a "single element" mentality. It remains difficult to generalize a single metric across populations due to the variations in individual preferences, decision-makers, circumstances, and situations.[26,42,57,60,61] Whether we look only at clinical outcomes or economic outcomes, we must realize that several elements play a role in decision-making, regardless of the decision-maker's role or position.

Decision-makers should try to understand all perspectives (e.g., patients, clinicians, and payers) – as they are all involved in the decision-making process to one degree or another.[26,28,41,43,60-63] Every decision has a ripple effect on another perspective.

What goes into clinical and economic-driven decision-making?

Clinical Decisions

Many clinicians focus on data regarding safety and efficacy to make clinical decisions – with less attention on cost. Examples of questions asked for clinical outcomes centric decisions include:[1,29,64,65]

- What is the most clinically appropriate medication for this patient to achieve the desired health outcome?
- What procedure or service (irrespective of cost) will help the patient achieve the maximum health benefit?

Many clinicians are unaware of the cost of many products or services unless they make a conscious effort to acquire this information or it was conveyed to them by patients or other providers.

Economic Decisions

Questions of cost often come into play and can have a significant impact on healthcare decision-making. Examples of questions asked for economic outcomes centric decisions include:[1,66-72]

- Is the product (e.g., medication) or service (e.g., a medical procedure) covered under the patient's insurance?
- What is the cost of the medication to the health system and the patient?
- What is the cheapest medication available to the patient?
- How much is the institution saving by providing a particular product or service?

Traditionally, decision-makers calculate the acquisition costs of a product (e.g., medication) and include it with the clinical assessment to demonstrate its value.[73] However, total costs do not just stop at the cost of the medication. Assessing cost implications using acquisition costs of drug therapies is a narrow and unreflective approach to evaluating the economic impact of a treatment or service.[1] There are other associated costs with every sequence of events in an individual's life, including those related to health consequences.[28,40] Chapter 7 provides numerous cost items included when evaluating the economic burden of a product or service.

The aim of many individuals, institutions, and systems is to reduce healthcare costs. Therefore, economic data must be incorporated into the assessment of value and decision-making, along with the other clinical and safety endpoints.

Both Clinical and Economic Decisions

Examples of situations that use both clinical and economic decisions include:[1,29,42,54,57,67-71,74]

- Controlling prescribing behavior – e.g., through the use of a formulary or a drug list. For formulary decisions, clinicians often consider the cost. Medication formulary decisions at both individual, institution level, and nationally have to consider what to add or remove from the list continuously. They answer questions such as:
  - Should medication be added or removed from the formulary?
  - What are the cost and clinical implications of adding or removing a drug from the formulary?
- Coverage and reimbursement decisions. Should we reimburse for this product or service?

- Evaluation of a new service (e.g., clinical pharmacy services). Should we implement a new service? What is the value of this new service concerning the clinical outcomes and cost savings? If the service costs more, is the added benefit worth the additional cost?

One should evaluate both clinical and economic choices when a decision has to be made between options due to limited financial resources. Use both clinical and economic decisions to make a decision based on the benefits and costs.

Decision Questions

When deciding between two or more agents or services, it is crucial to identify your **decision question**.

Are you deciding:
- Which agent is more clinically effective? For example, does it lead to improved health – e.g., improved survival, QOL?
- Will this product or service allow you to reach your goal or the goal of those you serve?
- Is this new product or service appropriate, and to whom?
- Is the added benefit of a product or service worth the added cost? It depends on whom you ask.
- Which product or service costs less?
- Which product or service results in cost-savings (irrespective of clinical outcomes)?
- Should I (we) reimburse for this product or service?
- Should I (we) include a drug on the formulary?
- Should I (we) add or remove a service?

Decision Criteria

Several factors play a role in decision-making. Each individual and organization may identify and place varying priorities on these factors. A few factors that can influence healthcare resource allocation decisions and are often integrated into the decision-making process include:[5,11,20,29,42,53,75,76]

- Equity, fairness, and compassion
- Public health benefit
- Epidemiological
- Medical
- Legal considerations
- Ethical
- Cultural and social values
- Economic analyses, such as pharmacoeconomic (PE) analyses*

*Anyone who ultimately has the power to make any decision in healthcare needs to equip themselves with the skills to conduct or, at the very least, evaluate outcomes research, of which PE is a type. Outcomes Research (OR) has become the foundation for providing the evidence to measure quality, identifying potentially effective strategies, and making informed decisions to improve value and quality of care.[7,43,84] PE is a subset of health economics that focuses on pharmaceutical interventions.[1,29,53] PE is used to inform resource allocation decisions and define effective pharmaceutical policies.[1,25,29,53,73,88] PE analyses should only be one factor in the decision-making process. The use of PE as the only criterion is very controversial and not recommended. Different individuals or organizations determine the willingness to pay (WTP) threshold for quality-adjusted life years (QALYs) differently and use different cost-effectiveness (CE) thresholds to make a decision. Outcomes research and pharmacoeconomics are introduced and discussed in more detail, starting from Chapter 2.

It is challenging to combine numerous elements of value into a single metric for individuals that can further be effectively extrapolated to a population.[20,42,53] Decide what goes into your **decision criteria**. You will notice that this process is often more than just choosing the option that maximizes health benefits.

Decision-Makers

There are several decision-makers in healthcare. They vary in preferences, needs, authority, and impact on the decision question and context. Often, those with significant influence in practice are the clinicians and payers.

Start by asking, who are the decision-makers? It is essential to recognize that the decision-makers may not always be the ones benefiting from the decision.[26]

Examples of various stakeholders include:[1,9,25,26,29,62,73,74,77-81]
- **Health System Decision-makers or Administrators**: Chief pharmacy officers, directors of pharmacy, executives, and managers, due to their role in drug evaluation review, determine the potential value of new treatments, choose between alternatives, and provide general administrative responsibility across the healthcare system.
- **Clinicians in practice**: Individual healthcare providers (e.g., physicians, pharmacists, nurses) and trainees who evaluate literature to make and enforce clinical decisions.
- **Pharmacy and Therapeutics (P&T) committee members**: Due to their role in drug evaluation review and determining the potential value of new treatments.
- **Payers**: Health plans, medical groups, insurers, pharmacy benefits management (PBM) groups responsible for plan design.
- **Industry leaders**: Executives, administrators, and researchers at pharmaceutical companies, manufacturing facilities, and supply chain constituents.
- **Public health officials**: Individuals responsible for program development and evaluation.
- **Patients:** Individuals who need and/or receive care.
- **National policymakers:** Government entities (federal agencies) or national associations with policy-related activities, e.g., Centers for Medicare and Medicaid Services (CMS) and the Food and Drug Administration (FDA).
- **National and international organizations**: Organizations such as the National Committee for Quality Assurance (NCQA), the Joint Commission, and the World Health Organization (WHO).

Other more non-traditional decision-makers include:
- Editors from medical and outcomes research journals.
- Academic institutions[74, 77]
  - Academia: Deans, chairs, department heads, and faculty that use this information in educational curriculum design, research, or policy work in this area.
- Residency and Fellowship programs: Faculty, residents, and fellows. Particularly programs focused on managed care, drug information, and health administration.
- Researchers and analysts: Individuals who conduct the analyses determine what data to use, the best practices, and guidelines.

Consider using a decision-making questionnaire (such as the one shown in this chapter) to identify, clearly articulate, and understand your decision-making process.

Decision-Making Questionnaire

Evaluate your current decision-making process. Understand your environment and the criteria you use to make decisions. This questionnaire includes questions to consider when you are evaluating your decision-making process. Consider answering the questions in as much detail and honesty as possible. Be sure to note the perspective by which you are answering these questions. For example, are you answering the questions as the payer, provider of the health service (e.g., hospital or doctor), or patient?

The first step is to identify what you already do.

Needs Assessment

- What is your strategy for identifying your current and future needs?

- What is deemed critical to potentially sustain business as usual – i.e., your day-to-day items such as infrastructure and personnel?

- Determine what is relevant to your environment. What are your goals? What measures are pertinent to your situation?

Where do you currently spend your budget?

- Outline where you're spending occurs. For example, does it go towards infrastructure, personnel, medications, medical devices, equipment, technology, and hospital services? What you include should reflect the realities on the ground and not be a distorted "cleaner" or oversimplification of reality.

- What are your costly interventions?

- Where do you distribute your money?

- How do you prioritize your budget?

- What are you paying for? Is it worth it for you? If you pay for something, you expect an outcome. Is it creating enough value to justify its existence?

- What are the benefits?

- The benefit is to whom, and when will they see it?

- What has or will demonstrate the highest value? What other items do you think will add value?

- How do you assign your budget for healthcare personnel?

What are you willing to spend?

- What are you willing to pay for? To solve what problem?

- How much are you willing to pay to save a life or extend life for a year?

Decision-Makers

- Who are the decision-makers? For example, are they the clinicians or healthcare professionals (who have a significant influence on clinical decisions), the payer, patients, or shared decision-making across the various individuals (between the patient and clinician, patient, and health systems, among others)?

- Are those making the decisions paying for it? If so, they may be the ones most concerned with managing costs.

Decision-Making Process

- How do you make decisions?

- How and why would you choose one competing alternative or intervention over the other?

- Are your decision questions clear and easy to answer?

- Are the decisions time-sensitive? When does the decision have to be made? For example, immediately? End of day? End of the week? Month? Quarter? Year?

- Why is this even a question? Is the decision not obvious? For example, is one intervention more effective but also costs more?

- Are the decisions you make objective or subjective?

- How are you incorporating evidence into patient care and decision-making?

- What process does your organization take to determine where to allocate or invest?

- Are you allocating resources based on utilization?

- What systems or approaches are you using to prioritize and de-prioritize items?

- How emotionally invested are you in the decision question? When you are emotionally invested, you may become less objective and critical. We often pay for items we do not deem cost-effective but are the right thing to do. Do you use (or should you use) an objective outcome measure to determine the right thing to do?

<u>Value</u>

- Are you ranking based on value? If so, how are you defining value?

- What is the value, and to whom is the benefit going?

- What metrics do you measure for value and progress? Are you prioritizing these metrics? If not, why?

- Are you getting value for your money? This is necessary to answer when resources are low.

- As you continue spending money, are outcomes improving, staying the same, or getting worse?

- What are your warning signs for decreased value?

Decision Criteria

- Are you looking beyond efficacy, safety, and acquisition costs? If so, what are you assessing?

- Do you evaluate cost-effectiveness?

- What are your measures of effectiveness?

- What do you take into consideration when making a decision?

- What are your decision criteria? Check all that apply below. A few factors that can influence health resource allocation decisions and are often integrated into the decision-making process include:[5,11,20,29,42,53,75,76]
  - Equity, fairness, and compassion
  - Public health benefit
  - Epidemiological
  - Medical
  - Legal considerations
  - Ethical
  - Cultural and social values
  - Pharmacoeconomics (PE) analyses

Up Next

In this chapter, we discussed the scarcity and allocation of resources, realities on the ground compared with our goals, defining and focusing on value, and lastly, the topic of decision-making. A decision-making questionnaire was introduced to help you identify, clearly articulate, and understand your decision-making process. Consider using the empty pages at the end of the book to record the answers to the questions. In the next chapter, we will review a healthcare – innovation – outcomes (HIO) triad, outcomes research (OR), the difference between efficacy and effectiveness, and using evidence in real-world decision-making.

CHAPTER 2: A FOCUS ON OUTCOMES

Healthcare – Innovation – Outcomes (HIO) Triad

As we begin to dig deeper, consider focusing on healthcare, innovation, and outcomes collectively or using the **Healthcare – Innovation – Outcomes (HIO) Triad** to assist in broadly conceptualizing elements. Your goal is to make more objective, informed decisions and achieve the best value for your money.

Healthcare

The healthcare space is complex and ever-changing. Healthcare systems involve multiple practice settings (e.g., inpatient, outpatient, long-term care), practice disciplines (e.g., pharmacy, medicine, nursing, public health), numerous provider types, and of course, encompasses multiple products and services. Evaluate what products and services you currently use and your strategy moving forward (e.g., expansion or reduction of products and services provided).

Innovation

There is a desire and drive for innovation across sectors, particularly in healthcare. We work to redesign the care coordination process to optimize individuals' roles to deliver collaborative, team-based, patient-centered care. Where do you and your organization fall on your commitment to innovation? Is this reflected in your practices?

Curiosity drives innovation. Greater innovation allows for new products and services to be introduced to address a specific need. With these introductions, competition arises, and decisions must be made regarding optimal resource allocation. Each product or service competes with another that claims to add value. Innovation allows for greater competition, and competition allows for greater innovation.

Innovation can come at a price. When new innovative products and services come to market, you should ask: is the innovation adding or replacing anything in current practice? If it is replacing, you should consider determining the cost-effectiveness of this innovation compared with current methods or standards of care. Doing this allows you to determine the benefits associated with new interventions relative to existing practices.

Essential questions to ask when assessing the new options are:
- Is the added benefit worth the additional cost?
- What effects does this have on healthcare delivery?

Some decision-makers may invest in interventions that add value and decrease their spending on those interventions with higher value replacements. While this may be tricky in healthcare, the premise is the same.

In any discipline, we ask, is this innovation adding value to what currently exists?

Recognizing that new initiatives are costly and require capital investments, you should ask, what will it take for an organization to invest? How likely will your organization invest in new products or services, or interventions? Be able to answer: what process does your organization (or you) take to determine what and where to invest? You often have to evaluate the innovation and demonstrate its value to encourage investment.

Decision-makers and leaders are continually looking for ways to innovate and strategies to create value. Allocating resources to those products and services deemed to demonstrate higher value can positively influence sustainable, scalable innovation. Seek out and prioritize innovation where you have determined there is value. However, keep in mind that resources are limited – which means we may not be able to pay for everything that adds value at once or at all times.

Outcomes

To reach a goal of accelerating innovative transformation in healthcare, one should include and evaluate measurable outcomes. Outcomes include clinical, economic, and humanistic outcomes – you can find more on this on pages 43-44. Determine whether you are measuring or evaluating one or more of these outcomes to drive your decisions.

The traditional safety and efficacy endpoints are not enough to demonstrate the value of an intervention. Go beyond these measures and include data generated from real-world effectiveness evidence.[7,12,82,83] More on this can be found starting on page 45.

Outcomes Research

Outcomes Research (OR) has become the foundation for providing the evidence to measure quality, identifying potentially effective strategies, and making informed decisions to improve value and quality of care.[7,43,84] OR is a broad, complex, and holistic methodological discipline that aims to provide effectiveness data about the benefits, results, and real-world impact of interventions in practice.

According to the Agency for Healthcare Research and Quality (AHRQ), "Outcomes research seeks to understand the **end results of particular healthcare practices** and interventions. Outcomes research has altered the culture of clinical practice and healthcare research by changing how we assess the end result of health care services. For clinicians and patients, outcomes research provides evidence about benefits, risks, and results of treatments so they can make more informed decisions."[84]

OR focuses on the assessment (identification, measurement, and evaluation) of the end results of health interventions in real-world settings.[25,62,74,79,84] It addresses a broad spectrum of issues from individual patient-level treatment choices to macro-level questions that impact policies and regulations, financing, and delivery of care across health systems and countries.[74,79] It addresses the various interrelated outcome measures to help decision-makers determine which treatment or intervention to choose (and for whom) to achieve the best outcome.[79]

We often ask ourselves:
How do you integrate measures to determine "benefit" or "effectiveness"?

Assessing the end result of an intervention requires integrating and consolidating many different outcomes. Outcome measures are multifaceted and multivariate. They form the basis for improving healthcare and public health. Outcomes are "probability statements" and require integrating and consolidating many different components. OR also measures how people function and their experience with care. Final outcome measures may take time to develop; therefore, intermediate outcomes are often needed and measured.[1,2,9,12, 25,26,29,43,44,54,73-80,86-88]

Chapter 2: A Focus on Outcomes

To evaluate the true value of a product or intervention out in practice, all applicable outcome measures that determine its true effectiveness need to be considered. Therefore, OR goes beyond clinical outcomes to include humanistic and economic outcomes.[74]

The field of OR is continuously growing. There is a need for health professionals to be at the forefront of identifying and implementing multidisciplinary interventions and programs of quality and assessing the impact of healthcare interventions on the patient care experience.[79] More research is needed to identify policies that increase access, reduce costs, and improve health outcomes.

Performing Outcomes Research

Common groups of individuals who perform OR include:[1,2,12,25,26,29,43,44,54,73-79,86-90,99]
- Clinicians – e.g., physicians, pharmacists, and nurses
- Academic institutions – e.g., faculty and staff
- Researchers, healthcare analysts, and others – e.g., sociologists, biostatisticians, and epidemiologists
- Economists
- Health Systems – e.g., decision-makers within the institutions
- Payers – e.g., health plans, medical groups, pharmacy benefits management (PBM) groups
- Policymakers, public and private agencies
- Pharmaceutical companies.

Reviewing and Using Outcomes Research

OR is used in various settings and by different disciplines. It can be used and read by all the decision-makers outlined in Chapter 1.

OR can be used in:[1,2,12,25,26,29,43,44,54,67-80,86-91,99]
- Formulary management process
- Treatment guidelines
- Disease state management programs
- Coverage decisions
- Quality improvement initiatives
- Deciding on services to implement or replace

- Creating institutional and national policies and practices. It can help shape, support, and drive decisions (from micro to macro scale).[80]

Some agencies (e.g., National Committee for Quality Assurance [NCQA] and the Joint Commission) require outcomes evaluations to demonstrate the achievement of health goals and outcomes.[80]

Any decision-makers' goal is to make more informed decisions, considering benefits, risk, patient preferences, and experiences in addition to the clinical results of treatment and services. Recognizing that the actual effectiveness of a treatment or intervention depends on factors that are both clinical and non-clinical, OR looks to evaluate the impact of a product or service on clinical, economic, and humanistic outcomes.[79] It evaluates measures that are important to patients and sheds light on how patients experience care.[84]

Several outcome measures are used in OR to demonstrate the value of products & services.

To demonstrate the value of new products and services, one can track and monitor one or all three of these outcomes: economic, clinical, and humanistic. The Economic, Clinical, and Humanistic Outcomes (ECHO) model is frequently mentioned in the literature and encompasses these three outcomes.[25,74,92]

Clinical Measures

Clinical measures are objective physiological measures (e.g., blood pressure, body mass index, cholesterol levels, heart rate), morbidity, mortality, disease prevention, and complication rates, which are used to summarize changes in health outcomes. Clinical outcomes are often obtained through laboratory tests, physician assessments, and clinical events to assess the impact on health status.[1,43,73,74,79]

Clinical studies focus on safety and efficacy as the primary measures of interest. However, the clinical effectiveness of an intervention is impacted by other measures.[1] Clinical measures are the most common outcome measure and are used in comparative clinical effectiveness research to evaluate the effectiveness, benefits, successes, and failures of various treatment options available to inform decision-making.[1,80,97] There is a need to go beyond clinical measures to measure the impact and effectiveness of interventions in the real-world.[7,94-96]

OR provides a realistic picture of the realities on the ground that impact the success or effectiveness of interventions. Evaluating the true result of an intervention goes beyond merely assessing specific clinical markers to determine the success of an intervention. OR has allowed us to better evaluate and measure the quality of care.

Humanistic Measures

Humanistic measures are subjective measures used to assess the impact of a disease or intervention on patient-reported measures, such as quality of life (QOL), patient's health status, patient preferences, health perceptions, patient satisfaction, symptom reports, and functioning well-being. These measures are used to complement clinical outcomes of physical health and are obtained using surveys and questionnaires, such as health-related quality of life (HRQOL).[29,43,74,79,98]

Economic Measures

Economic measures are the costs relevant to an intervention. These include direct medical costs and non-medical costs, as well as indirect costs of healthcare.[1,25,29,42-44,53,73,98-101] These measures are assessed using economic and **pharmacoeconomic (PE)** analyses such as cost-effectiveness analysis (CEA), cost-minimization analysis (CMA), and cost-utility analysis (CUA). Incorporating economic measures with clinical and humanistic outcomes helps make more informed administrative decisions influenced by cost and budget restrictions.[80]

Efficacy or Effectiveness?

The drug approval process in the United States (US) is dependent on safety and efficacy data.[12,83,102-104] Decision-makers often use efficacy data to extrapolate effectiveness – since effectiveness data is not always available. However, uncertainty remains between efficacy in the lab and effectiveness outcomes in the real-world.

Decision-makers should recognize the limitations of relying on and generalizing efficacy data in practice. It is essential always to question the limitations of the data presented to you. There is a gap between evidence generated from efficacy data compared with effectiveness data in practice. A drug that may be efficacious in a randomized controlled trial may not be deemed as effective in clinical practice.[1,74,105,108] The type of data presented to you, whether its efficacy or effectiveness data, must be noted.

Let's start with differentiating between efficacy and effectiveness.

Efficacy: Controlled Environment

The "efficacy" of the product is established to determine if a product works or if it can work under ideal and controlled conditions.[1,29,73,74,105]

Randomized control trials are used in Phase I to III studies to assess the safety and efficacy of products in small, homogenous populations under ideal, controlled environments using specific regulated and standardized study protocols. While these methods allow for high internal validity, these restrictions limit the generalizability of the efficacy data to larger populations.[1,26,29,73,102]

Effectiveness: Real-World Environment

Healthcare decision-makers are interested in knowing whether a drug works for those it was studied to treat in real-world settings to make more informed decisions of its value out in practice. To do so, they need to evaluate effectiveness research.[1,7,12,25,26,29,43,73,74,94,95,103-107] Comparative effectiveness research (CER) is widely used to inform decision-making in practice.[26,43,80,97] Effectiveness measures can be determined through the use of post-marketing observational studies, Phase IV studies, and patient registries in larger, more heterogeneous patient populations.[1,29,43,73,74,105] Evaluation of practices in the real-world allows for higher external validity compared with the evaluation of these practices in controlled settings. However, these studies often lack control groups – which is a major limitation of this approach.

OR is considered effectiveness research and not efficacy research.

Questions you will need to answer when reviewing data are:
- Is the evidence generated from a controlled setting or real-world practice?
- What are the limitations of the data you have?
- Why do you need the data?

Decision-makers would like to rely on more real-world data (RWD).[7,94,103,104] The Food and Drug Administration (FDA) defined RWD as "the data relating to patient health status and/or the delivery of health care routinely collected from a variety of sources."[96,109] As for real-world evidence (RWE), it is defined by FDA as " clinical evidence regarding the usage and potential benefits or risks of a medical product derived from analysis of RWD."[96,109] We are moving beyond safety and efficacy to include RWD within our databases and use that data to inform our decision-making process better (in practice, clinical trial design, drug development, and regulation).[18,96,103,109] The FDA provides guidance and frameworks for the use of RWD and RWE for drugs, biologics, and medical devices to assist with regulatory decision-making (e.g., drug approvals).[96,103,104,110,111]

Using Evidence in Real-World Decision-Making

New information is generated all the time. We are continuously implementing new initiatives, such as new products, service lines, and patient services, to improve health outcomes, convenience, quality, and reduce costs.[7,13,59] These initiatives all generate data that will help further inform decision-making in healthcare. How we ultimately evaluate and use the data determines the usefulness of this information in practice.

Leverage the data and evidence of the past and present to make better-informed decisions for the future. We have come to find out that our experiences are incorporated into our decision-making, and the sources of knowledge – where we get our information from – can influence or lead to variations in treatment.[2,26,112] We have shifted our efforts to include RWD within our databases, out in practice, and use that evidence to better inform our decision-making process.[1,2,7,25,26,66,94,95,108,113-115]

The key is to continuously strive for data-driven strategies.

We are regularly asked to assess if and how we can use the data in real-world settings. Often new data, evidence, or knowledge are generated and published for others to read and use. However, a publication-to-practice gap remains. There is a gap between the new data and evidence produced and incorporating it into practice and decision-making.[26,112,116]

Decision-making in healthcare is often time-sensitive.[112] However, it can sometimes take evidence years to ultimately be used and applied into practice. The time to incorporate or use the new data, evidence, or knowledge in practice can increase or decrease based on many elements.

Elements that Influence Time

Four main elements can influence the time to use or incorporate new data or evidence into practice. The elements and factors that impact the time of utilization in practice are summarized below. The arrows mean the following:
- ↓: decrease time to use or incorporate the data or evidence in real-world practice. Faster uptake of the data or evidence.
- ↑: increase time to use or incorporate the data or evidence in real-world practice. Slower uptake of the data or evidence.

Chapter 2: A Focus on Outcomes

Element 1: The Data or Evidence

Factors associated with the data or evidence element that influence time include:

A. *Applicability of the information in that practice.*

Is the new information generalizable to the practice? Are the populations similar? How applicable or generalizable is it to the population in practice?

Examples:
- ↓ time/faster uptake: increased applicability in that practice or patient population leads to less time to use.
- ↑ time/slower uptake: not applicable to the patient population or practice.

B. *Quality and source of the evidence.*

Examples:
- ↓ time/faster uptake: high quality of data and evidence. The comfort level of the user with a decision increases when the quality of the evidence is high.
- ↑ time/slower uptake: poor quality of data and evidence. The comfort level of the user with a decision decreases when the quality of the evidence is low.

C. *Impact of the information or perceived impact or value "size" of the new knowledge in practice. How "big of a deal" is it? Urgency driven: how important or critical is the information?*

Examples:
- ↓ time/faster uptake: high impact – it can or will alter care. For example, new practice guidelines that change practice or drugs recalled for safety issues have a faster uptake time.
- ↑ time/slower uptake: small interventions (maybe too specialized or are not done frequently) with limited evidence may take longer to incorporate.

Element 2: The Institution

Factors associated with the Institution element that influence time include:

A. *Frequency of review and update of policies, procedures, and formularies.*

How often are these regularly updated? Continuous vs. episodic updates and management?

Examples:
- ↓ time/faster uptake: policies, procedures, and formularies are regularly reviewed and updated.
- ↑ time/slower uptake: policies, procedures, and formularies are not regularly reviewed and updated.

B. *Resources available to the institutions.*

Are institutions able to obtain the most updated information? How fast can information resources be acquired? For example, more resources are available more quickly in large academic centers compared with independent, smaller community or private institutions.

Examples:
- ↓ time/faster uptake: frequent and easy access to the latest information.
- ↑ time/slower uptake: limited access to the latest information.

C. *Execution on that information and changing processes based on recommendations.*

The complexity of the process to incorporate new data. For example, the complexity of the information technology system when changes need to be made (e.g., infrastructure issues). What processes are in place or what platform(s) are available – to share, deploy, and learn new information?

Examples:
- ↓ time/faster uptake: Minimal or limited process changes or obstacles.
- ↑ time/slower uptake: Several obstacles in place and process changes required.

Element 3: The Individual

Factors associated with the Individual element that influence time include:

A. *Training of the professionals in literature review, pharmacoeconomics and outcomes research (PEOR), and evaluating evidence.*

Examples:
- ↓ time/faster uptake: Highly trained or well-versed professionals in literature review and critique of the literature (e.g., often read and utilize new studies in updating practice recommendations).

Chapter 2: A Focus on Outcomes

- ↑ time/slower uptake: Personnel not trained (or limited training) in evaluating literature appropriately.

B. *Decision-making process.*

Examples:
- ↓ time/faster uptake: Individual(s) use their own clinical judgment in conjunction with data.
- ↑ time/slower uptake: Individual(s) prefer to use their own clinical judgment or experiences with little reliance on new data.

Element 4: Both the Institution and Individual

Factors associated with both institution and individual element that influence time include:

A. *Ease of incorporating it into practice.*

How easy is it to integrate into practice?

Examples:
- ↓ time/faster uptake: Easy (or easier) to incorporate it into practice – requires minimal changes.
- ↑ time/slower uptake: More challenging to incorporate due to time, expense, and lack of expertise.

B. *Availability of information.*

How fast can they obtain the information?

Examples:
- ↓ time/faster uptake: Easy (or easier) access to new data for both institution and provider.
- ↑ time/slower uptake: Limited access to that data (i.e., if an institution or practitioner cannot access the information) – new data is simply unable to be read, assessed, and incorporated.

C. *Execution on that information and changing processes based on recommendations.*

The complexity of the process to incorporate new data. The complexity of the information technology system when one needs to make changes (infrastructure). What processes are in place or what platform(s) are available – to share, deploy, and learn new information?

Examples:
- ↓ time/faster uptake: Limited process changes or obstacles.
- ↑ time/slower uptake: Several obstacles in place and process changes required.

D. *Culture around change and the use of evidence-based medicine or evidence-based decision-making.*

Previous experience in introducing change.

Examples:
- ↓time/faster uptake: Culture is strong and sees great value in incorporating the latest evidence.
- ↑ time/slower uptake: Culture is weak. Less likely to change if you do not see value in evidence-based decision-making.

E. *Reliance on scientific knowledge to drive behavior.*

Is the institution or professional guideline-driven or authority-driven?

Examples:
- ↓ time/faster uptake: Relies on scientific knowledge to drive behavior. This can also be in addition to their own clinical judgments and experiences and a combination of other sources of knowledge; however, scientific knowledge is of high importance.
- ↑ time/slower uptake: Relies on other sources of knowledge used in that practice setting (e.g., tradition, authority, trial and error, and logical reasoning).[112]

Each of the elements and the associated items influence time to clinical implementation differently. The presence of one or more elements can vary depending on the institution, environment, or a combination of factors. "Implementation science" or "implementation research" involves strategies for evaluating and facilitating the utilization of data and research into practice to improve health services and outcomes.[116,117] It moves beyond efficacy and effectiveness research and looks at items such as exploration, acceptability, adoption, implementation, appropriateness, sustainability.[116,117]

Up Next

In this chapter, we discussed a healthcare – innovation – outcomes (HIO) triad, what is outcomes research, the difference between efficacy and effectiveness, and using evidence in real-world decision-making. In the next chapter, we will introduce the basics of pharmacoeconomics (PE) and examine the significance, rise, and limitations.

CHAPTER 3: PHARMACOECONOMICS

Basics of Health Economics

As in other sectors, healthcare requires tradeoffs, and choices must be made due to resource limitations and conditions of scarcity.[2,43,118] Traditional evaluations of products or services that many clinicians are familiar with focus on clinical outcomes. However, decisions are also often based on costs and can have far-reaching financial implications.

Health economics bridges between economics and healthcare to evaluate the supply and demand of healthcare resources – and assess the impact on the population as a result.[1,29,118] Economic evaluations are only a few decades old and go beyond the clinical measures – those often used to evaluate the consequence of an intervention – to include items such as costs and patient preferences.[43,73]

There are several types of economic evaluations, and they differ in the measurement and valuation of the consequences of health interventions.[2,119,139] Economic assessments and evaluations have a prime seat on the table when making healthcare decisions.

What is Pharmacoeconomics (PE)?

Pharmaceutical products and services are associated with significant economic expenses in the healthcare sector and society as a whole.[13,30,35,36,86] The total prescription spending in the US is estimated to have reached $476 billion in 2018.[36] We cannot cut out the cost associated with manufacturing, distributing, administering, and dispensing medications from our budgets. Until we create another medical intervention more powerful than medications to prevent and treat disease, medications will continue to be an integral part of healthcare delivery. Decision-makers need to be judicious in allocating their resources to enhance the use of pharmacy products and services and manage rising costs to optimize patient outcomes.

Once you add economic measures to clinical or humanistic measures in an analysis of pharmaceutical interventions, it becomes a **pharmacoeconomics (PE)** study.[29,44,73]

PE is a type of outcomes research (OR) and a subset of health economics that focuses on pharmaceutical interventions.[1,29,53,120] The goal of PE is similar to OR – it is used to inform decisions of resource allocation within institutions. PE "identifies, measures, and compares the costs and consequences of the use of pharmaceutical products and services"[1,25,29,73] to inform resource allocation decisions and define effective pharmaceutical policies.[53,88]

PE highlights both the costs and outcomes of products and services together. PE merges cost analyses with clinical and humanistic data. This method allows decision-makers to evaluate both the costs and patient health outcomes to estimate the value of a pharmaceutical product or service.[29,44,53] It assesses the input costs consumed to produce the outcome or consequence (clinical, humanistic, or economic effects) of the product, service, or intervention.[1,29,44,73] PE helps answer the question: "is the added benefit of one pharmaceutical product or service worth its added cost?"[29,53] PE fills the gap of evidence and information to assist with efficiently allocating these scarce resources.

Overall, in PE analyses, you will:[1,25,29,44,53,73]
1. **Identify** choices or competing alternatives – e.g., new medication vs. standard of care or a new pharmacy service vs. no pharmacy service. At least two competing choices are optimal.
2. Recognize the metrics that will be **measured** to evaluate the outcomes and costs.
3. **Compare** both the costs and outcomes of the choices or options.
4. **Decide** or recommend between the options.

Significance & Rise of Pharmacoeconomics

The field of PE is only a few decades old, first appearing in the literature around 1986.[29,73] Greater attention has been placed on the field since then, as the number of published PE analyses have amplified, and the methodologies have advanced.[2,26]

PE analyses are increasingly being incorporated into the decision-making process due to the need to objectively assess the competitive options available under conditions of limited resources (resource scarcity), budget constraints, high costs, and an increased number of options for individuals and populations.[1,73,81,121,122] It is believed that incorporating PE will enhance value to patients, providers, institutions, the payer, and ultimately the health system at large.[28] Patient-level to national-level decision-makers utilize the output provided by these evaluations to compare the total costs of the interventions and their associated benefits to manage budget constraints and respond to the question of value.[26,29,42]

During allocation decisions, providers are continually being asked: what value does this product or service provide? The demand to conduct and understand PE analyses has grown out of the need and pressure faced by decision-makers and health care providers to quantify and justify the value of the products and services available or provided.[1,73] One can consider applying the PE principles in practice to assist with identifying cost containment strategies to help manage rising costs. Healthcare professionals need to equip themselves with the skills to conduct and evaluate PE studies.

While you may not be conducting PE, all healthcare professionals need to understand, interpret, and critically evaluate PE literature. Such abilities will assist them in translating the results of the analyses into practice and determining its relevance in healthcare decision-making.[26,29,121]

Role of PE Analyses in Decision-Making

It is often recommended that decision-makers use a transparent, streamlined, intentional approach to choosing between available options.[7,26,29,42,63,123,124] Information generated from PE analyses may be used to make decisions on a patient-by-patient basis as well as determine national policies on a global (macro) scale.[29,88,125]

PE analyses play a role in the evaluation of drug products and services and are used as a tool to assist in managed care, drug benefit design, coverage policies (including policies on step-therapy, prior authorization), making medication formulary management decisions, drug pricing decisions, and developing drug use and treatment guidelines and disease management programs.[1,26,29,44,73,86,122]

PE can be used to answer questions such as:[1,29,42,44,54,74,88]
- Should we add or remove a medication from the formulary?
- What are the cost and clinical implications of adding or removing a drug from the formulary?
- Should we reimburse for this product or service?
- Should we implement a new service? What is the value of this new service with regards to clinical outcomes and cost savings? If the service costs more, is the added benefit worth the additional cost?

Medication Formulary Decisions

Health systems, hospitals, and health plans all periodically review their drug formularies. Some incorporate information provided from PE analyses and PE methods to streamline and inform their medication formulary decisions.[1,25,29,54,63,73,86,121-126]

Guidance from organizations such as the American Managed Care Pharmacy (AMCP) on formulary submission for review by health plans highlights the inclusion of economic information along with the safety and efficacy information of medications.[29,74,80,85]

If you work in a hospital or health system, evaluate what economic information is included in your reviews and assess the gaps and quality of the evidence. For example, your Pharmacy and Therapeutics (P&T) Committee may review documents for the addition or removal of medications and, therefore, may evaluate the cost of medications and any costs associated with administering the medications.

Incorporating PE into Decision-Making

As part of the Decision-Making Questionnaire (Chapter 1), go back and answer the following:
- Are you looking beyond efficacy, safety, and acquisition costs? If so, what are you assessing?
- Do you evaluate cost-effectiveness?

Cost-Effectiveness

The phrase "cost-effectiveness" is too often misused and is considered subjective when stated without further clarification. When someone tells you that something is deemed cost-effective, the first question that should come to mind is what is it measured against to be considered cost-effective? That is, the intervention or product is cost-effective compared to what intervention or product? What are we comparing it to? For something to be cost-effective, it must be measured as more cost-effective than a comparator or an alternative option (more cost-effective compared with an alternative option). It is a ratio; therefore, there needs to be two groups.

Everyone has a different threshold for how they define cost-effective.

The standard approach used worldwide to measure and summarize the value of a healthcare intervention (product and service) among outcomes researchers is the **cost-effectiveness analysis (CEA)**.[9,20,21,40-42,45,49,122] This approach uses an incremental cost per the measure of health gain – often quality-adjusted life years (QALYs) – to join both value and cost in a single metric. How patients value health outcomes is an integral element and should be an item of concern for both payers and clinicians. Hence, the importance of using measures such as QALYs – which is discussed later.

Starting Point

Gaps in evidence exist to inform decision-making objectively. CEAs are often used as a starting point in the decision-making process to understand the long-term value.[5,11,19,20,29,42,45,53,75,76] CEA sheds light and provides evidence on the population effects of new or existing therapies, programs, tests, and interventions to assist decision-makers in comparing the value of these options to allocate resources to those that fit their needs judiciously.[77,99] CEA allows you to compare existing products and services to innovation to deliberately address questions of where to invest your resources.[42]

Criticism with CEA is based on the premise that we cannot possibly combine all the elements that go into the valuation of something in a single metric. Due to the heterogeneity of individual preferences and value definitions (i.e., individual variation in value criteria), it is complicated and difficult to combine numerous elements of value into a single metric for individuals – especially one that can also be effectively extrapolated to a population.[7,20,26,41,42,57]

The cost-per-QALY metric of CEA is recommended as a starting point and is a core component of value assessment used to inform discussions in health plans coverage debates.[9,41,42] While PE analyses, specifically CEA, can be used to inform a decision, they should not be used as the only decision criteria item – but rather, one of many.[53,75] It is recommended to use CEA as an aid alongside other decision criteria determined by individuals or institutions.

Start by defining the **decision criteria**.[42] For a list of factors that may influence health resource allocation decisions and are often integrated into the decision-making process, see Chapter 1. Decide what goes into your decision criteria. You will notice that it includes more than maximizing health benefits.

Global Perspectives and Use in Decision-Making

The use of PE analyses to inform national drug approvals, pricing and formulary decision questions in healthcare is common outside of the US.[1,7,26,29,54,88,129-132] The diverse strategies depend on the country, their health systems in place, and are tailored to individual needs.[7,54,133]

Issues with the Use of PE Analyses

Within the healthcare setting, professionals often have to make decisions quickly, especially regarding immediate patient care. There is a need for real-time information tools that help improve decision-making. However, the use of PE analyses in daily decision-making among health professionals remains limited.[121] Although we have witnessed trends toward increased use of CEA, it also has experienced criticism.

Major Limitations of Pharmacoeconomic Analyses

The limited uptake of PE analyses into daily operations is due to several internal and external factors that act as roadblocks to applying this information in real-world practice.[7,9,11,26-29,44,57,60,87,115,121,131,134-138]

These factors include:[7,9,11,26-29,44,57,60,87,115,121,131,134-138]

- Time
- Resources – lack of resources internally and or externally
- Lack of training and expertise
- Cost
- Availability of reliable information
- Generalizability
- Skepticism of the literature
- Bias
- Complexity of the analyses
- Lack of transparency
- The use of a single metric to assess value
- Quality of reported economic evaluation and the magnitude of benefit varies considerably by study
- Publication-to-practice gap
- Other considerations in the decision-making process: e.g., ethical considerations, culture, and political factors around "rationing."

Let's discuss a few of these limitations in a little more detail.

Time. The approach to the decision-making process may vary based on whether the decisions are immediate, daily, short-term, or long-term. Time urgency can determine how much information we can obtain and use for our decision-making process. Due to the face-paced nature of healthcare environments, decisions must be made – and options are chosen – regardless of whether PE data is available.

Availability of reliable information. Retrieving PE data from internal or external sources is dependent on the availability of the information. Even if data are found, they may be incomplete. Also, there are not enough PE analyses to answer all decision questions.

Generalizability. There are issues with translating available PE information to the appropriate practice setting. Issues arise when attempting to convert the findings to unique real-world settings.[7,28,137] Economic analyses focus on a specific population for whom the analysis was performed and do not reflect that population's diversity. While there are standards and validated decision aids, limitations still exist due to the uncertainty that remains with how all individual-level variations are aggregated and incorporated.[20,26,41,42,121,138,139]

Quality of reported economic evaluation and the magnitude of benefit varies considerably by study. An example of this is extrapolating data from short-term studies to make a decision(s) that can impact patients and the institution long-term. There are limitations to this approach.

Publication-to-practice gap. Determine whether the recommendation(s) will reach the right people at the right time or if there is a difference between when the information is available and when implemented in practice.

If or when conducting PE analyses internally (or in-house), you should also consider infrastructure and cost.

- *Infrastructure:* Evaluate whether the institution has the support necessary to perform or evaluate PE analyses. There is no internal peer-review process at some institutions to provide a critical evaluation of the methodology of PE analyses.
- *Cost:* There are several costs associated with conducting the research in-house. These are costs related to the time and resources involved in the process of collecting, obtaining, and evaluating the data.

These factors should be acknowledged and addressed to assist with applying and disseminating PE analyses to the appropriate target audiences.[28]

How We Learn Pharmacoeconomics

While the topics of PE, OR, and evidence-based medicine are within core competencies and curriculums in professional programs (e.g., pharmacy, medical schools, and public health), we need to do more to ensure all healthcare professionals have the basic working knowledge of the fundamentals of PE.[1,29,140-152]

Traditional training methods remain limited and have failed to reach everyone. These have included training in the classroom setting, textbooks, additional graduate-level degrees (masters or doctorates), and postgraduate training (residencies and fellowships). However, with all of these methods, there continues to be a lack of expertise and training in this field. Historically, the ideas and methods of the discipline are presented the same way – in the form of textbooks that read the same style and contain the same information. There is a need to see the "world of pharmacoeconomics" in all its facets from a macro-level. This means understanding what it would take to perform and evaluate these types of analyses (from the content to the teams and ultimately communicating the information).

Agencies, such as the Academy of Managed Care Pharmacy (AMCP), Agency for Healthcare Research and Quality (AHRQ), The Professional Society for Health Economics and Outcomes Research (ISPOR), National Pharmaceutical Council (among many others) provide additional resources to assist in educating professionals on PE analyses and OR.[19,20,55,62,74,85,97,120,127]

Up Next

In this chapter, we discussed basic health economics, the definition, significance, rise, and limitations of PE. In the next chapter, we will introduce and discuss the various types of PE analyses.

CHAPTER 4: ECONOMICS ANALYSES

Overview of Economic Analyses

The four main types of analyses used in pharmacoeconomics (PE) to inform decision-making include cost-minimization analysis (CMA), cost-benefit analysis (CBA), cost-effectiveness analysis (CEA) and cost-utility analysis (CUA).[1,2,9,25,29,43,44,53,73,98,153,154] Other types of analyses include cost-of-illness (COI), cost-consequence analysis (CCA), budget impact, and marginal analyses.[1,20,29,42-44,73,87,139,156]

You may find multiple types of analyses within one evaluation or study (e.g., a CEA and CBA in one study).[29,139] Each analysis differs in the **decision question**, **decision criteria**, costs, and outcome inputs used.

Figure 1 summarizes the costs, outcomes, measures associated with each type of analysis. Start on the left side of the figure and ask:
* Are the outcomes of interest deemed to be equivalent?
* How do you measure the outcome of interest?

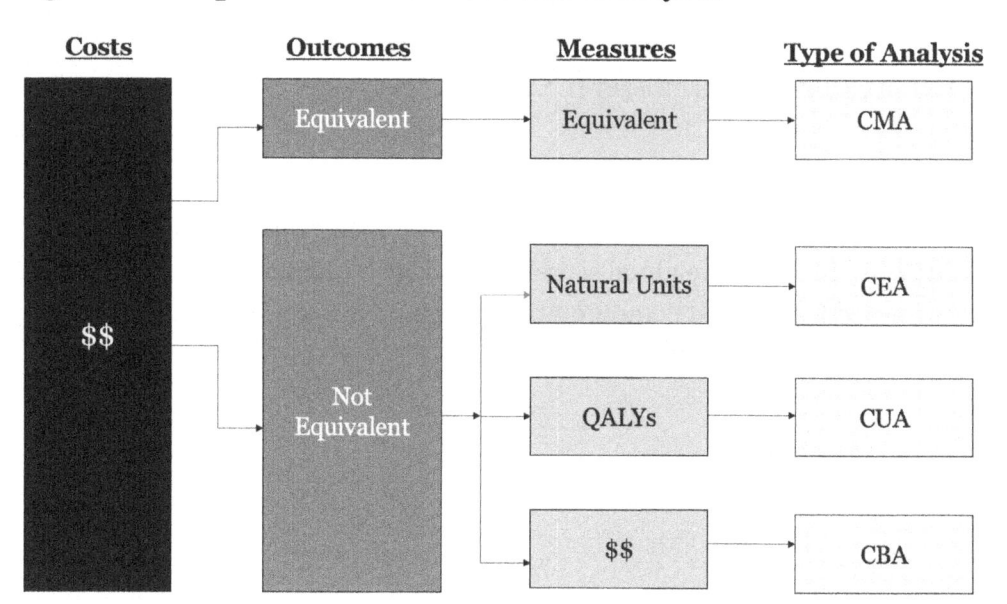

Figure 1: Comparison Across Economic Analyses

Costs	Outcomes	Measures	Type of Analysis
$$	Equivalent	Equivalent	CMA
$$	Not Equivalent	Natural Units	CEA
$$	Not Equivalent	QALYs	CUA
$$	Not Equivalent	$$	CBA

$$ = dollars or any monetary value; QALYs = quality-adjusted life years; CMA = cost-minimization analysis; CEA = cost-effectiveness analysis; CBA = cost-benefit analysis; CUA = cost-utility analysis [1,2,25,39,43,44,53,73,98,153]

A study is considered just a "cost analysis" or "partial analysis" when only the costs are included, and the associated outcomes or consequences are not incorporated or "measured" in the analysis.[25,29,157,158]

Examples of cost-analyses in the literature include:
- Patel and colleagues conducted a cost-analysis to examine the financial impact of Matrix-assisted laser desorption ionization-time of flight (MALDI-TOF) in combination with antimicrobial stewardship resources on total hospital costs.[157]
- Kaakeh and colleagues assessed the impact of drug shortages on U.S. health systems and evaluated the labor costs associated with managing drug shortages.[158]

Table 1: Overview of Economic Analyses

Costs
Consistent across all analyses – the input is costs in dollars or other monetary units.

Cost-minimization
Outcomes are assumed and or proven to be equivalent.

Cost-effectiveness
Outcomes are measured in natural units (e.g., years of life gained, blood pressure, lives saved, cures, blood glucose) and must be the same across all interventions or competing alternatives in the analysis. These are the outcome measures many clinicians are most accustomed to seeing in practice and ordinarily retrieve from clinical efficacy (i.e., clinical trials) and effectiveness studies.

Cost-utility
Outcomes are measured in utilities to incorporate subjective measures (e.g., quality of life) and patient preferences. Utility is defined as a weighted score from a scale ranging from 0 to 1, where 1 is "perfect health," and "0" is dead. The most common utility measure is a quality-adjusted life-year (QALYs) and is considered a preference-based measure.

Cost-benefit
Outcomes are measured in dollars or monetary units.

Sources: 1,2,25,29,43,44,53,73,98,153,154

Cost-Minimization Analysis

Cost-minimization analysis (CMA) compares the costs and consequences of at least two interventions with equivalent outcomes.[1,25,29,43,44,73,153]

Examples of CMA include:
- Comparison of brand versus generic version of the same drug with confirmed equivalency[1,29,43,73]
- Comparison of two generics of the same drug with confirmed equivalency[29,43]

This analysis is the simplest to conduct, as it compares intervention with outcomes that are assumed to be equivalent and do not need to be measured. Therefore, costs are the only measures compared between interventions or competing alternatives.[1,25,29,44,53,73,153] However, consequences are still assessed in this analysis to confirm equivalence. The data supporting the equivalency must be stated and evaluated appropriately.[73,139]

Examples of CMA in the literature include:
- Neel and colleagues conducted a CMA to compare immediate sequential cataract surgery and delayed sequential cataract surgery since they noted that both demonstrated similar safety and efficacy profiles.[159]
- Davis and colleagues conducted a CMA to compare total laryngectomy and postoperative radiotherapy versus organ preservation in the treatment of advanced laryngeal cancer since both demonstrated similar survival rates.[160]
- Men and colleagues conducted a CMA to compare amisulpride and olanzapine in schizophrenia treatment in China since systematic reviews demonstrated similar efficacy of the two agents.[161]

CMA is used to determine the least costly option among interventions with comparable benefits or effectiveness, as the decision favors the lowest total cost option or intervention.[1,29,73,153]

Decision criteria = choose the least costly option.[73]

Again, once the equivalence of outcomes is confirmed, only costs are compared between interventions to make a decision. Results are summarized as the average cost per patient.[73]

Table 2: Cost-Minimization Analysis (CMA)

Advantages
- Simplest to conduct.
- Used when products or services have equal outcome measures of interest (such as safety, efficacy, and effectiveness outcomes). An example includes generic versus its branded medication.
- Outcome measures are deemed equivalent, therefore, are not measured.
- Only costs are compared among competing options.
- **Decision**: The decision favors the lowest total cost option.

Disadvantages
- The quality of the analysis depends on the quality of the evidence that supports outcome equivalence. This is consistent with all quality data.
- Criticism among researchers with the use of this analysis: if it only measures costs and not outcomes, is it a full PE analysis?
- Often, the simplicity of this analysis does not reflect the realities on the ground.

Cannot use this analysis if:
- Outcomes are not equivalent (e.g., the brand and generic should be FDA rated equivalent). Any differences in outcomes between the products or services no longer permits you to use this analysis.
- Outcomes of competing options are different.
- Compare different classes of medication or different disease states.

Sources: 1,25,29,43,44,53,73,153

Cost-Benefit Analysis

Cost-benefit analysis (CBA) is used to estimate the benefit of an intervention and is distinct from the other analyses since both the costs and outcomes (or "benefits") are expressed in monetary terms.[1,2,25,29,43,44,53,73,77,99,139]

Converting the consequences or outcomes that result from an intervention to monetary units (or their deemed financial equivalent) allows the decision-maker to compare costs and benefits of multiple diverse interventions or programs for the same or completely different diseases – regardless of any other clinical and humanistic measures.[1,2,29,43,73,153] For example, conditions with different health outcome measures such as asthma and diabetes.[1,2,29,43,73,153] This allows for decisions to be made between programs – e.g., will you fund a bicycle helmet program or fund a program for stroke prevention? Depending on the decision-maker and the scope or breadth of the decisions they are required to make, many consider using CBAs to compare interventions or programs across different sectors.[1,73] If you have a portfolio of interventions you have to choose from, you may consider a CBA. Remember, the same outcomes (dollar [$] or a monetary value) are measured across different programs, which permits comparison across various interventions, diseases, and sectors.

These comparisons cannot be done with other analyses, such as CEA or CUA, which require the same outcome measure type and are dependent on the disease or intervention.

As a decision-maker, you care to know:
- Are the benefits of implementing an intervention greater than its costs?
- How does this intervention compare with other interventions or programs that are part of the choices?

CBA allows decision-makers to assess whether the benefit (expressed as a monetary value) exceeds the costs of implementation – and by how much.[1,2,29,44,153] This assists decision-makers to choose the intervention with the highest net benefit.

For example, Caro and colleagues conducted a CBA to compare implantable cardioverter-defibrillator (ICD) versus amiodarone for primary prevention of sudden cardiac deaths in patients with heart failure in the UK and France from a health-care system perspective.[162]

Decision Criteria

The results of a CBA are calculations of net benefit and the benefit-to-cost or cost-to-benefit ratios. Net benefit (net benefit = benefits – costs) is calculated and expressed as a sum.

The decision is made when:
- If the net benefit is greater than zero, then on an individual level, that intervention is financially viable.[1,2,43,73] When the choice is between implementing a program or not (the "with or "without" approach), the choice of implementing or choosing the program becomes easy when net benefits > 0. But when we evaluate the net benefit from a societal perspective and assess its societal benefit, we may choose the intervention(s) or program(s) that have a negative net benefit due to values or causes of equity and social justice.[29,153] We are often unable to fund every intervention or program that demonstrates a positive net benefit due to limited resources and budgets. Therefore, the next decision is made by choosing between interventions to maximize the return on investment – with preference to the program or intervention with the highest net benefit or choosing between the highest benefit-to-cost ratio.[1,2,73]

Desired is a net benefit > 0, a benefit-to-cost ratio greater than 1:1 and a cost-to-benefit ratio less than 1:1.[2,43,73]

Methods

The three main approaches used in the monetary valuation of outcomes in CBAs include the human capital (market valuation), willingness-to-pay (stated preference), and revealed preferences.[1,73] Refer to additional resources for more information on the details of each method. Whichever one you use can determine what decision you make, as they may not always lead to the same conclusion or decision.[73] Articulate which approach you used and what the limitations of using each method.

Table 3: Cost-Benefit Analysis (CBA)

Advantages
- Allows the comparison of costs and benefits across multiple diverse interventions or programs for the same or completely different diseases.
- Easier than CEA and CUA to make a decision based on the results, as the **decision criteria** and **rule(s)** are pretty straightforward.
- **Decision:** Desired is a net benefit > 0, a benefit-to-cost ratio greater than 1:1 and a cost-to-benefit ratio less than 1:1.[2,43,73]

Disadvantages
- Difficulty associated with placing a monetary value on a benefit (e.g., how productive are you or how much do you contribute to society?) is a primary concern of CBAs.
- The variety of methods of measuring and valuing benefits and lack of a standard agreement on how to place a monetary value on benefit has led to imprecise and dissimilar estimates across analyses.

Sources: 1,2,29,43,44,73,153

Cost-Effectiveness Analysis

Cost-effectiveness analysis (CEA) is the most popular of the analyses and is used when there is a proven clinical (and/or statistical) difference between the interventions in question.[21,43,73,87,153] It is used when we would like to know how one intervention compares to another in terms of costs and effectiveness.[9,29,53,86]

CEA is used as a tool to help determine the value for the money spent.[2,41,43,44,73,125] The outcome measures remain as they were collected – as natural health unit and are not converted to a monetary value.[1,2,29,139] Providers are very familiar with the natural health units, both in clinical practice and in the efficacy and effectiveness literature, and therefore, may consider it the most relevant to them.[29,98]

CEAs are only used to <u>compare two or more interventions</u> and programs with the same outcome measure, such as natural health units or life-years saved.[2,9,29,43,53,98,131]

CEA cannot be used to compare the cost-effectiveness (CE) of interventions with different clinical units. For example, you cannot compare the CE of implementing an asthma program with implementing a cholesterol management service due to differences in outcome measures used to demonstrate value (e.g., forced expiratory volume [FEV] measures versus serum cholesterol levels).[1,2,29,73]

CE is measured as a **ratio** (cost per effectiveness) since it assesses the cost-effectiveness of a product or service compared to another choice or a competing alternative.[1,9,42,73,77,98]

Incremental Cost-Effectiveness Ratio

An incremental cost-effectiveness ratio (ICER) is used to evaluate what intervention provides better outcomes for the smallest costs.[2,73,131] It assesses the change in cost divided by the change in effectiveness or outcome of two competing alternatives.[1,9,29,43,44,77,87,98,131] ICER represents the cost per one extra unit of effectiveness.[138]

If the ICER is negative, it means that one strategy is either more costly and less effective (**dominated** strategy, reject this option), and the other strategy is more effective and costs less (**dominant** strategy, accept this option as cost-effective).[1,2,29,43,98] **A dominant strategy is considered cost-effective**. A negative ICER is not calculated or reported, but rather one would either indicate that the strategy was dominant or dominated.[1,2,21,29,43,73,98,125]

An ICER would be relevant to calculate in a situation where one option is more effective than the other; however, it also costs more than the second option – and therefore, would result in a positive ICER.[29,43] In this case, one would like to assess the added cost per unit of effectiveness of health benefit to determine whether the additional benefit is worth the extra cost.[1,2,29,43,73,98] Institution have varying willingness to pay threshold that they use to determine if they consider this strategy cost-effective based on the ICER obtained.[1]

Cost-Effectiveness Plane

To visually compare the alternatives, one can use a cost-effectiveness (CE) plane.[2,29,43,73]

Box: 1

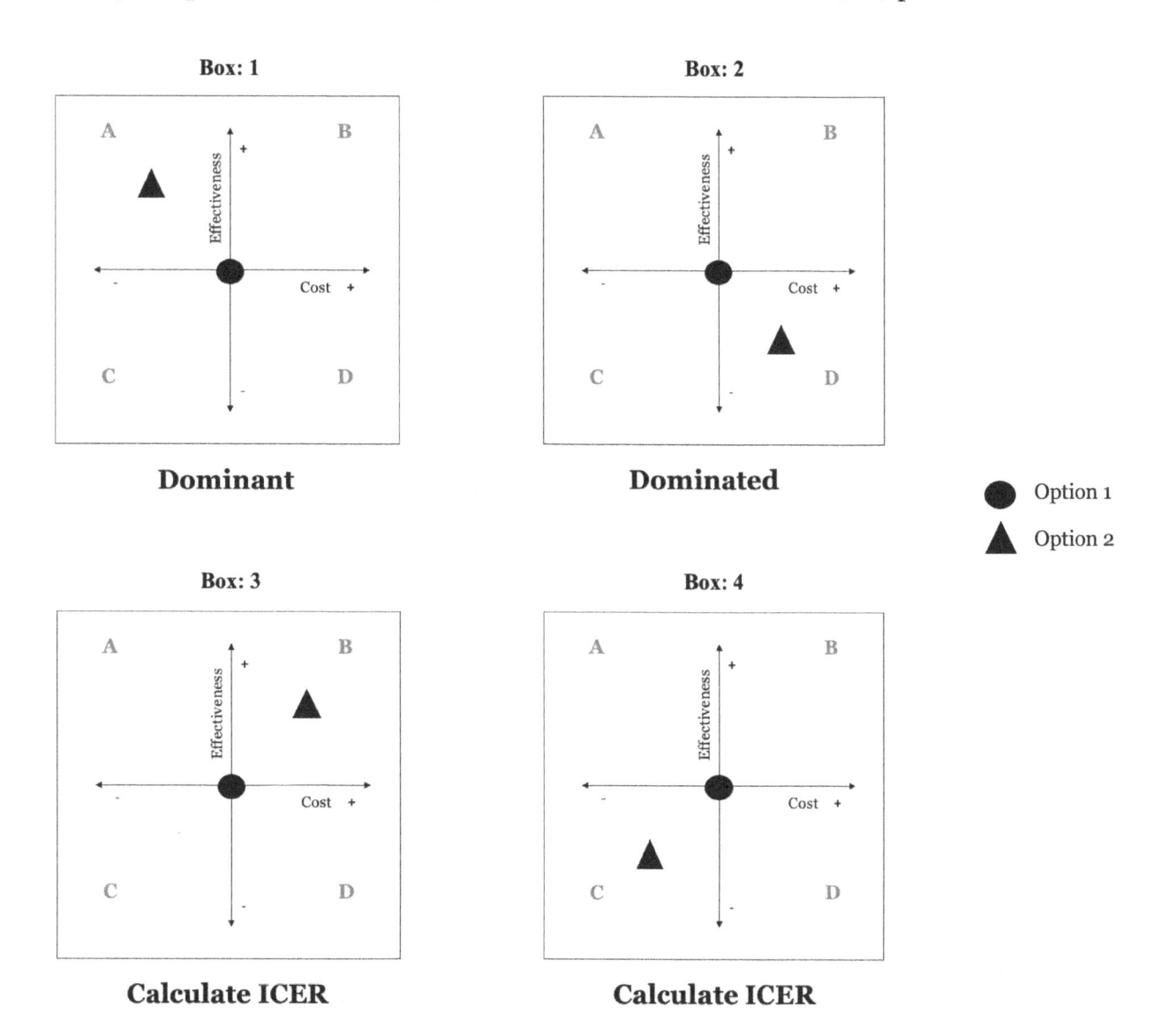

Dominant

Box: 2

Dominated

● Option 1
▲ Option 2

Box: 3

Calculate ICER

Box: 4

Calculate ICER

71

In the figures, we are comparing option 2 (new) to option 1 (standard of care, which is now called the "standard comparator") on the plane. In the middle, you will find option 1 indicated. The x-axis is cost, with the right side being increase or higher cost and the left side being decrease or lower cost. The y-axis is a measure of effectiveness, with the top half being greater effectiveness and the bottom half being lower effectiveness.

Box 1: If option 2 is more effective and costs less than option 1, then it is considered the **dominant** strategy, and the decision-maker would accept this option as cost-effective.[2,9,29,98]

Box 2: If option 2 is either more costly and less effective than option 1, it is considered the **dominated** strategy, and the decision-maker would reject this option as it is not cost-effective.[2,9,29]

Box 3 and 4: A decision-maker would have to make a decision when an option falls in one of the two quadrants (B and C), where option 2 is either more effective but costs more or is less effective but also costs less. An ICER should be calculated for these quadrants.[2,29,44,73]

Decision Criteria

The measure of effectiveness is based on <u>one</u> outcome measure, which is the same across interventions or competing alternatives.[2,73,86,98] The decision-maker is left to evaluate how other factors, not included in the final assessment, impact the results.

The decision that results from this analysis is hard to make. The decision criteria are based on a judgment call: one needs to decide if the extra unit of effectiveness is worth the additional cost and does not incorporate other items that the decision-maker or patient may value.[21,29,73]

As a decision-maker (or anyone assessing whether a product or service is cost-effective), you should answer the following questions:
- What is the product, service, or intervention measured against to be deemed cost-effective? That is, the intervention is cost-effective compared to what? What are we comparing it to? Remember, it must always be compared to something.
- What value would you place to deem something cost-effective? That is, would you consider the added cost worth the added gain in effectiveness? Do you have a cutoff point? Are you using a threshold?

There is much variety in CEA – you may hear, "If you have seen one CEA, you have seen one CEA." Each CEA can look quite different.[29,153]

Examples of CEA in the literature include:
- Najafzadeh and colleagues conducted a CEA of novel regimens for the treatment of hepatitis C virus since the new agents appear more efficacious yet more costly.[163]
- Prabhu and colleagues conducted a CEA comparing Descemet stripping automated endothelial keratoplasty (DSAEK) and penetrating keratoplasty (PK) for corneal endothelial disease in the United States (US) adults.[164]
- Kaakeh and colleagues conducted a CEA of three health system-wide HMG-CoA reductase inhibitors (statins) sample policies in post-myocardial infarction patients over age 65 years of age.[165]

Table 4: Cost-Effectiveness Analysis (CEA)

Advantages
- Most popular of the analyses.
- The outcome measures remain as they were collected – as natural health unit and are not converted to a monetary value.
- Providers are very familiar with the natural health units – in clinical practice and both efficacy and effectiveness literature.

Disadvantages
- Only used to compare interventions and programs with the same outcome measure or endpoint or clinical unit.
- Each CEA looks different.
- The measure of effectiveness is based on <u>one</u> outcome measure for all interventions evaluated. The decision-maker is left to assess how other factors, not included in the final assessment, impact the results.
- The **decision** that results from this analysis is hard to make. The decision criteria are based on a judgment call: decide if the extra unit of effectiveness is worth the additional cost.
- The data used in the analysis is taken from population averages and does not account for patient heterogeneity.

<u>Cannot</u> use this analysis if:
- Outcomes of products, services, or interventions are different.
- Compare different classes of medication or different disease states.

Sources: 1,2,26,29,41,43,44,73,98,153

Cost-Utility Analysis

Cost-utility analysis (CUA), a subtype of CEA, is identical to CEA in terms of costs, but the effectiveness measure is quality-adjusted life years (QALYs) rather than other natural health units.[1,2,40,43,44,53,73] CUAs are often called cost-effectiveness analyses.

In CUA, the outcomes are measured in utilities to incorporate subjective measures (e.g., quality of life) and patient preferences. Utility is defined as a weighted score of various health states from a scale ranging from 0 to 1, where 1 is "perfect health," and "0" is dead.[2,9,29,44,53,73,77,99,128,153] A higher utility number means the more preferable the outcome.[98]

The most common utility measure is QALYs and is considered a preference-based measure.[1,2,9,40,44,53,73,138] QALY takes into account that states of health before death are not all the same. Some medical care can increase the length of life without improving the quality of life (QOL). In some cases, QOL is "reduced" in hopes to lengthen life (e.g., chemotherapy).[2,29,53,153] CUA is summarized as the cost per QALY gained.[1]

If you see a CEA with the ICER denominator used being QALYs, then it is a CUA. The ICER ratio is similar to CEA except that it is only the change in cost over the change in QALYs: **CUA ratio = Δ cost/Δ QALYs**.[1,2,40,44,73]

Examples of CUA in the literature:
- Baumann and colleagues conducted a CUA comparing internet-based cognitive behavioral therapy (ICBT) to face-to-face cognitive behavioral therapy (FCBT) in Unipolar Depression.[166]
- Wateska and colleagues conducted a CEA of five pneumococcal vaccination strategies in US adults aged 65 years or older.[167]

Decision Rule

The conventional approach or "central method" is to use the cost-per-QALY metric for a **cost-effectiveness threshold**.[42,45,77,99,128,156] The threshold range often seen in the literature is the $50,000 to $150,000/QALY is not based on any rigorous analysis.[45,73,156] Several analyses may not provide decision criteria or explicitly state whether they are using a threshold in the decision-making process.

Various methods exist to determine QALYS and health-related quality of life and include visual analog scales, rating scale, standard gamble, and time trade-off.[1,29,44,73,98,154] Refer to additional resources for more information on the details of each method. Make sure to note what method was used in any CUA analysis you conduct or evaluate and determine whether it was appropriate.

Generic and disease-specific instruments are health-related quality of life preference-based utility instruments commonly used to evaluate domains of physical, social, the general perception of health, disease-specific functioning, mental health, and emotional well-being.[1,44,53,98]

Examples of generic instruments include:[1,2,29,43,44,53,73,77,98,99,153]
- Short-form 36 (SF-36)
- EuroQol 5D (EQ-5D)
- European Quality of Life Index (EQLS)
- Quality of Well-Being Scale (QWB)
- Years of Health Life (YHL)

Disease-specific instruments include:[1,53,98]
- Asthma Quality of Life Questionnaire
- Diabetes Quality of Life Questionnaire

Numerous methods and tools exist to calculate preference and health status measures. Consider seeking additional information on the quality of life assessments, health-related quality of life, patient-reported outcomes measures, and methodology for all.

If you would like a list of CUA analyses published, Tufts Medical Center for the Evaluation of Value and Risk in Health overseas, a CEA registry of over 8,000 cost-utility analyses published from 1976 to 2018 is available online.[49,168]

Table 5: Cost-Utility Analysis (CUA)

Advantages
- Subset of CEA.
- Combines morbidity (quality of life), mortality (quantity of life), and different health outcomes into a one-unit measure.
- Expresses improvement in cost per quality-adjusted life-years (QALYs) gained. The cost per QALY takes into account the state of health during each year of life.
- Incorporates patient preferences – measured in terms of utility (QALY).
- Uses a value-weighted index of health to evaluate improvement.

Disadvantages
- No consensus on the best method to measure utility weights, although many methods exist.
- Requires the use of a valid instrument to gauge patient preferences.
- Debate continues over how well QALYs truly reflect patient preferences. Therefore, carefully critique and interpret it with caution.
- It requires time and resources to conduct and collect the data for this analysis.
- The **decision** that results from this analysis is hard to make.

Sources: 1,2,29,40,42-45,53,73,77,98,99,125,153,154

Other Types: Cost of Illness

A cost of illness (COI) analysis, also referred to as burden-of-illness analysis, is calculated and used to determine and compare the total economic burden of disease states on society (e.g., the financial burden of heart disease).[29,43,44,53,73]

COI analyses attach a total healthcare cost to a disease state to emphasize the magnitude of resources required and the cost burden of that disease state. COI analyses are used primarily for advocacy and political reasons to aid in shifting allocation decisions to treatment and prevention programs in disease states with substantial economic burdens.[29,73] While it serves to shed light on the burden of the disease, it does not give guidance on how to allocate the costs to achieve efficiency and value.[29,153]

COI analyses are not used to compare medication treatments but rather to examine the economic burden of one disease state compared to another (e.g., cost of epilepsy versus breast cancer) and potentially the same disease across different location (e.g., cost of diabetes in Chicago versus the cost of diabetes in Paris).[29,43,73]

COI analyses vary from other PE analyses in that outcomes are not assessed.[43,73] The methodology for COI analyses are not consistent, as there is no agreed-upon standard, and decision-makers are often left to make many assumptions.[29,43,153] Due to inconsistency in methods and lack of transparency in what costs were used, where they came from, and how they were calculated, a wide range of estimates can be found for the same disease state.[1,29,153] For example, COI analyses have been conducted to estimate the economic burden of pediatric anxiety disorders, maternal morbidity, and ischemic and non-traumatic hemorrhagic stroke.[169-171]

Other Types: Cost Consequence Analysis

A cost consequence analysis (CCA) does not attempt to compare interventions with a single measure or calculation but rather merely lists all costs and assorted consequences (a matrix of outcomes in natural units or utilities) separately in a disaggregated structure.[29,43,73,87,139] For example, Reimer and colleagues conducted a CCA to compare mobile stroke units versus standard transport to comprehensive stroke centers.[172]

There is greater transparency in CCA compared with COI in what went into the calculations (as it lists all costs estimated), and one can evaluate the comprehensiveness of the lists. The decision-maker is required to select the costs and outcomes that best match their perspective and decision question and then uniquely determine the value. CCA requires more work from the decision-maker.[43,73,153]

Other Types: Budget Impact Analysis

Budget impact analysis is an assessment of the budget use and impact for various stakeholders (e.g., health system, institution, insurance plans).[20,42,44,53,87,156] Budget impact analyses are not considered by some organizations a measure of value but rather a measure of resource use.[19,20,42] For example, McMullen and colleagues conducted a budget analysis to assess the impact of adding recombinant FVIII Therapy (for Hemophilia A) to formulary on the budget of US private payers.[173]

The information generated from budget impact analyses has been offered with CEA data to help inform decisions (e.g., formulary decisions).[1,174] However, various stakeholders and recommendations do not recommend the budget impact analysis alone as an integral part of value assessment.[20,42,156]

Up Next

In this chapter, we discussed the various types of PE analyses. In the next section, we will review designing, conducting, and evaluating PE analyses in three chapters. It includes Chapter 5: Designing and Curating the Experience, Chapter 6: Building the Team, and Chapter 7: The PE Canvas.

SECTION 2: DESIGNING, CONDUCTING, AND EVALUATING PHARMACOECONOMICS ANALYSES

Section 2: Designing, Conducting, Evaluating

LIFECYCLE

The Lifecycle of a PE Analysis

Five major building blocks:
1. Design
2. Execution or Implementation
3. Evaluation or Assessment
4. Communication
5. Decision

DESIGN & BUILD

Design and Build the PE Base

Four pillars of the PE Base:
1. Need
2. Individuals
3. Value
4. The Process

THE PROCESS

DOMAINS

Domains of The Process
1. Environment
2. Time
3. Study Components
4. The Team

The Process illustrates four major domains and seven essential elements required to conduct and/or evaluate PE analyses.

ELEMENTS

Elements of The Process
1. Defining Standards
2. Organization
3. Designing and Re-designing
4. Execution or Implementation
5. Evaluation or Assessment
6. Communication Strategies
7. Implementation Strategies and Processes after Completion

PE = pharmacoeconomics

CHAPTER 5: DESIGNING AND CURATING THE EXPERIENCE

Researchers are Designers

The healthcare sector continues to see intensive transformations driven by new models of care and initiatives. What drives many healthcare decision-makers to be creative is their desire to find new ways to achieve the best outcomes for patients.

In healthcare, we are already designing new products and services to address unmet needs and achieve target outcomes. The overarching goal is to design cost-conscious interventions that add value and improve health outcomes. Much like we design our practice sites, new programs, and new products, we should design how we demonstrate the value of the products and services. There is a need to focus on how we create value and how we tell our "value" stories. This calls for an add-on to our existing design processes to ensure the demonstration of "success" and value. To continuously add sustainable and scalable value in healthcare, professionals need to be creative, innovative, patient-centric, and outcomes-driven individuals.

The process to design, create, implement, demonstrate, evaluate, and communicate value is a **design process**. Be intentional in designing value. When you design or perform a new intervention, you need to build in the systems to demonstrate its value. We need those working in healthcare to broaden and evolve their skill sets to move beyond merely describing these new interventions, initiatives, products, or services – but also to be able to evaluate and articulate the value to diverse stakeholders.

As we work to foster innovation in healthcare, we should see ourselves as designers – designing products, services and demonstrating and communicating the value. As you get ready to introduce, perform an intervention or initiative, or conduct research – **have a designer mindset.** Suppose we treat what we design as a piece of art, our desire to be creative and innovate increases. When we design anything, we have a responsibility to embed innovation and design thinking.

Chapter 5: Designing and Curating the Experience

To systematically answer a decision question and use an evidence-based approach, a decision-maker should **consider using a researcher's mindset and strategies**. Therefore, decision-makers are referred to as researchers in the next section. Researchers may also be called "designers" or "creators" throughout the book.

Researchers are designers, and designers are researchers.

How are designers and researchers similar? Well, both:
- **Are visionaries**, innovators, and have a **maker's or creator's mindset**. Both have a culture centered on curiosity, creativity, innovation, and a willingness to try new things.
- Have a passion for designing, developing, and deploying. Both have a desire to create something from nothing, very little, or several items – even items that may seem unrelated.
- Believe **no two are the same**. No two original designs or art pieces are the same, and no two research projects or analyses are precisely the same. **Every study is different.**
- Immerse themselves with the **processes** and **outcomes** of designing new experiences.
- **Pull in expertise**, talent, funds, and feedback to create something.
- Have a clear idea of what they hope to achieve or test.
- **Create** something that answers a question, solves a problem, or tells a story.
- Track and **evaluate progress** made, **learn from mistakes** along the way, and **assess** whether the outcome met criteria or their standard.
- Their work requires **planning** and **forecasting**. Like many art pieces or designs, research requires time, discipline, and some level of **risk.**
- Have **patience**. They realize these things take time and are comfortable with this since they know where they are ultimately going.
- **Imagine the final product** and work their way back by taking small steps forward.
- Think big by also thinking small. Both see the final product or result and work back in small nugget sized pieces.
- Continuously focus on both the **big picture** and **small details** of the process and results.
- Know what their final product will be and how they will deliver their message. Both want to convey a specific message with what they create.

- Both require some level of **technical skills** based on the project they are pursuing.

Nevertheless, overall, both start with a blank canvas.

Research is an art form with multiple facets and processes. Each step – or stroke – along the way (either small or large) affects the final piece or result. Designers and researchers need a well-defined canvas and approach. Designers and Researchers both begin to fill a canvas with the skeleton, core elements, and domains of the work.

Like producing any form of art, there is a process that is valued and required to direct one to their intended result. To start "painting," designers and researchers need to identify all the necessary resources to get the desired product. We need the "physical" resources (e.g., paint, data, etc.), the talent (people), the time and commitment to perform such a task. Both take the time to adequately design a study or process to answer the research questions and effectively meet the needs.

Due to the analogy of a canvas, a **resource** was created to assist in creating and evaluating PE evaluations. The **Pharmacoeconomics (PE) Canvas** (Chapter 7) is meant to be used as a framework to begin to craft your strategy and find gaps and opportunities to learn and improve. Other tools, such as the Lifecycle of a Pharmacoeconomic (PE) Analysis, PE Base, Domains, and Elements of The Process, were also created in this Chapter to help you visualize all the different pieces included in these studies.

You are a designer – now craft the strategy.

It is essential to have a vision, be patient-centric, and results-driven when you design and craft your strategy to achieve better outcomes and provide greater value. Think like a designer from beginning to end to curate the experience and craft the facets of your plan. Design your research and evaluation methods for one that will assist you in crafting a value proposition. Design the solutions and the process to achieve results. Design, build and then execute the process.

Lifecycle of a Pharmacoeconomics Analysis

Before we get into the intricacies of the process, let us look at the entire process from a macro-level. Figure 1 is a broad bird's eye view of the lifecycle of a PE analysis. It is the journey of ideation to outcomes and, ultimately, the decision.

There are five major building blocks when it comes to the lifecycle of a PE analysis. The five building blocks include the design, execution, evaluation, communication, and decision. The individual building blocks will be discussed in more detail in other sections.

Five Building Block in the Lifecycle of a PE Analysis

- *Design*: Designing and creating the analysis.
- *Execution*: Executing or implementing the analysis.
- *Evaluation*: Assessing and synthesizing results – then framing recommendations.
- *Communication*: Communicating the methods, results, and recommendations.
- *Decision*: Making a decision.

The "action" of the user is at the end of the lifecycle. Answer the question, "Will the user act on this information?

Figure 1: Lifecycle of a Pharmacoeconomics Analysis

CREATION		DEMONSTRATE & COMMUNICATE		
DESIGN	**EXECUTE**	**EVALUATE**	**COMMUNICATE**	**DECIDE**
1. Identify the question you are trying to solve (the question at hand) and the competing alternatives.	3. Design the analysis.	6. Measure the output (data analysis).	8. Compare and propose recommendations (compare competing alternatives and propose recommendations).	9. Decide: make a decision with the information provided.
2. Compare the competing alternatives	4. Build the model and methods required.	7. Evaluate the results.	9. Decide: make a decision with the information provided.	10. Implementation strategy after or based on decision.
3. Design the analysis.	5. Conduct the analysis.	8. Compare and propose recommendations (compare competing alternatives and propose recommendations).		

Pharmacoeconomics Base

A critical initial component of any design is the "base" or "foundation" for which other elements will be added. In this section, we start by identifying the fundamental building blocks of the base or the foundation for PE analyses. PE analyses, particularly cost-effectiveness analysis (CEA) and cost-utility analysis (CUA) are multifactorial. Since there are many moving parts, it is necessary to have a strong base. Building the foundation for PE analyses requires clarity, simplicity, intentional, and strategic planning to appropriately execute and use of the information.

As you are designing and building an analysis, it is essential to **establish the conditions for success**. To help develop these conditions, focus on the following:
- Build the foundation or base for the analysis.
- Develop a basic set of skills, tools, practices, and an "idea synthesis" mindset. Combine ideas and perspectives from different professionals and disciplines to generate strategies.
- Recognize the build must be logical – it should make sense in practice and research.
- Reduce your own bias – do not come in with your personal bias of what works and what does not. Bring your expertise and experiences to add to the process and not influence the process.
- **If you ask better questions, you get better results.** Spend time asking and prioritizing the items you want to ask. The first step is to think in-depth about the most appropriate questions to ask to benefit from the answers. What do you want to answer? What are the relevant questions to ask to get these answers? The better the questions, the more useful your responses will be. Ask "what if" questions - not just "what" and "why."

Design and Build the PE Base

To appropriately build the PE Base, you need to think critically. You will build upon the base you create moving forward, thereby making this next section central to your strategy. Before starting to build and execute the analysis, **four pillars** are required to make the base or foundation and establish the conditions for success. The four pillars of the PE Base are **Need, Individuals, Value, and The Process.** These four pillars are meant to continually remind you and help you understand the direction you are going and the reason for it all. It is essential to bridge between these pillars – and to do so, communication among all those involved is vital.

Focus on these critical pillars by assessing and leveraging concepts of **knowledge and diversity** across each base pillar and throughout the analysis. Knowledge and diversity drive innovation creation.

Knowledge is identifying what currently exists and the knowledge you are adding with this analysis. It encompasses the information we know and the information we hope to achieve. It entails answering questions such as, what do we know? What do we still need to know? What do we know about our individuals throughout the process? These individuals can either be part of the team or part of the decision-making process, in general. Assess this for each pillar, domain, and item moving forward.

Diversity includes a diversity of stakeholders, environment, thought, and experiences. Diversity allows for higher idea generation and creativity in problem-solving and increased exposure to an assortment of audiences and impact streams. Everyone has a mosaic of characteristics that impact how they work and live. The innovation lies in how we position these unique characteristics and skills to add the most value.[50] Diversity also includes different products and services. Move past the term "it has always been done this way" and leverage diversity to create something new.

Four Pillars of the PE Base

Pillar 1. Need (or the Why)

Researchers, decision-makers, and analysts must identify **the need** and relevance of the information. To whom (or the audience) the analysis is conducted needs to be clear. Those performing and using the analysis have to understand the need for the decision question to assess its impact on their target population. Start by identifying the need for the analysis or the decision question. Do the necessary research to justify the rationale behind the study. This will enable you to speak to the need for such an evaluation.

It would be best to recognize the relevance or **why** you are evaluating these interventions to understand the use in practice. If you do all the work to conduct it, you should at least be sure you can use or benefit from the information generated. We need to move from insight into action. Do not just evaluate it; understand how you can use it. Consider creating a statement for what you hope to do with this information.

Why are we taking the time to answer this question? Identify the issue at hand and ask **why** is this question being evaluated?[25] How do you justify the reason(s) that this question exists? You need to set the stage for why the audience should care. Is this something they are likely to experience?

Evaluate how the need came about – e.g., was it a request? If so, start with the request and break it down. Have we identified an opportunity for which we need to decide? For example, a new medication is approved, and the Pharmacy and Therapeutics (P&T) Committee is now in charge of determining whether to add it to the formulary. How was the opportunity identified? You can either start with the question at hand or start with the population and then build a query around it. For example, you can focus on patients with diabetes and then formulate the question – or you can start with the question and then evaluate the population it affects.

Tell me what we know and tell me what we still need to know.

What is currently missing in the information that is out there? Where are the gaps? You must go one step further and ask, can the need be measured? **If you cannot measure it, you cannot manage it.** Were specific metrics used to formulate the question? If so, how will you include the parameter?

Next, determine when the information is needed. How quickly do you need the material? How fast do you need to make a decision? Also, determine whether the information and decision need to be delivered verbally or in written format?[25]

Pillar 2. Individuals

The individuals involved in the analyses and evaluation process are instrumental in the PE base and the lifecycle of PE analyses. They are vital to identifying and formulating the question, methods, analysis, and utilization of the information.

The "Individuals" referred throughout this section can be an actual person or an institution.

Start by answering the following questions:
- Who are the individuals involved in conducting and evaluating these analyses?
- Who are the beneficiaries of this information?

- Who are the decision-makers? Who are the individuals who are going to act on the insights developed from this analysis?

Now for each individual you have identified, answer the following questions:
- What is the role of each individual?
- What is their perspective?
- What power do they have and over what?
- What do you want them to do with that power? What would you like them to commit to doing?

There are three role categories for individuals, as shown in Figure 2:

Figure 2: Individuals

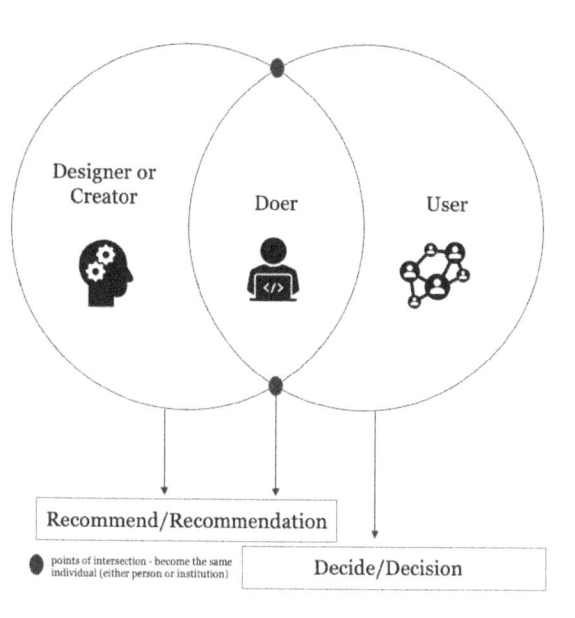

- **Designers/Creators**: Individuals who create or conduct the analyses and provide recommendations based on the results.
- **Users**: Individuals who use the information generated from the analyses to inform decision-making.
- **Doers**: Individuals who conduct the analyses and also use the information to inform decision-making. This individual is a combination of both the designer/creator and the user.

There are differences in the tasks or responsibilities of each of these roles; however, **all evaluate the literature**. It is imperative to identify who you are for a particular analysis. The functions often change depending on the question at hand, the specific analysis, or the audience since many individuals frequently switch between all three.

There are various ways each of these role categories communicates with each other – both internally and externally. Outline the communication streams and evaluate how each will communicate messages throughout the lifecycle. Gauge how each will deliver what they have achieved as a result of their roles.

Chapter 5: Designing and Curating the Experience

We are interested in how the user informs the designer/creator and doer and whether they apply the recommendations into practice. The process is a feedback loop.

For detailed information on the various backgrounds of the individuals involved in both conducting and evaluating PE analyses, see Chapter 6.

Designer or Creator

Blocks of the PE analysis to which they are involved:

1. Design
2. Execution or implementation
3. Evaluation or assessment
4. Communication

- **Identifies, measures, and compares** between interventions.
- Then **communicates results** and recommendations

There is no way a designer will be able to account for all the different decision contexts for all potential users.

Recommend

Doer

Blocks of the PE analysis to which they are involved:

1. Design
2. Execution or implementation
3. Evaluation or assessment
4. Communication
5. Decision

- **Identifies, measures, and compares** between interventions.
- Then **communicates results** and recommendations
- Then **decides** based on assessments.

Doers can design or conduct an analysis for the specific context for which they need to decide.

Recommend & Decide

User

Blocks of the PE analysis to which they are involved: Decisions

- They critically evaluate and assess all blocks to make a **decision**.
- Not actively involved in the creation of the other blocks but evaluate them to determine whether they can use this information.
- The action for the user is at the end.
- They answer the following questions: Will I or we use this information in decision-making?

There are differences in how the doers and users evaluate the literature. User evaluates its application on the ground within their population to answer, "Can this be applied to my particular case?"

Decide

Designer or Creator

- Researcher
- Individual creates and executes on the analysis – conducts the research and analysis

Can be either:

- In-house: at the institution that is asking the question – a closed system. Examples of in-house individuals in pharmaceutical companies, managed care organizations, P&T committees, hospitals, and governing bodies. Internal analyses may be conducted in an informal or formal and nonsystematic or systematic manner. It is highly dependent on the institution.
- External system: includes individuals that are evaluating it "from a distance." For example, individuals in academia conducting evaluations. In some cases, the creator (e.g., academic researcher) may not be in direct communication with the end-user or directly involved with the use of the information generated from the analysis. Academics conducting the research are often not the ultimate decision-makers and, therefore, have no direct influence on whether the results will be used in practice.

Doer (Designer and User)

- Researcher & Decision-maker
- Individual conducts, evaluates, and makes a decision.

The individual is both the designer and the user. They do the analysis and then do something with the information generated from the analysis. Doer can be both in-house individuals and other institutions or decision-making bodies that have resources to conduct assessments internally. Results may drive internal or external decisions.

User

- Decision-maker
- Individual decides whether they will use the data or evidence to inform a decision.

Users are often the target audience. These individuals were not involved in conducting the research, but instead, they evaluate the analysis and literature and decide if and how they will use it to inform decision-making. Usually, the analysis was conducted based on the perspectives of these individuals.

Chapter 5: Designing and Curating the Experience

Decision-makers may be present in any setting (in-house or external). They have the power to make a decision or influence decision-making. While many researchers may not be directly involved in the decision-making process in practice, they do make decisions on whether to use this information in their studies.

To help identify the users, answer the following questions:
- Who are the beneficiaries of this information?
- Who are the people who are going to act on the insights developed through this analysis?

Individuals – Decision-Makers

These decision-makers include those with significant influence on decision-making, such as clinicians or healthcare professionals, payers, patients, and government entities. There are times when there is shared decision-making between multiple individuals – like in the case of clinician and patient shared decision making.[62] For a full recap of various decision-makers, see Chapter 1.

Potential Challenges for Individuals

The challenges for all three role categories are similar to the limitation of PE analyses (see Chapter 3). Users frequently lack training in evaluating these analyses to apply to clinical practice, which remains a leading challenge. They are unfamiliar with the exact methods utilized by the designers and doers; therefore, they are unaware if they can appropriately generalize findings to their specific population of interest.

<u>Pillar 3. Value (What and to Whom)</u>

This section draws in your target audience – it is your message to the specific masses you are addressing.

Identify your target audience. The target audience may be those who will use the information generated from the evaluation (the primary decision-makers) or those who will potentially be impacted by the data generated.[77, 128] Tailor the analysis to the perspective of the ultimate end-user of the information.[40] Be sure to make it relevant to the target audience and decision contexts. Deliver what is important to the audience and perspective.

When thinking through your target audience, answer the following "Who" questions:
- Who benefits from or needs this information?
- Who will read this, and why?
- Who will it impact?

These may seem like the same question said in different ways; however, the answers may vary, so you are encouraged to answer each.

Define what value means to you, your organization, and then those of your target audience. Identify any perspective specific value metrics you used to define value – as these can differ between you and your target audience.

*Clearly state **what value is being created** and to **whom** with this analysis.*

What is the value proposition for the analysis? What is the value of answering the decision question? What is the benefit to the audience or reader, or user?

Answer the following questions to create a value proposition for the analysis:
- What is important to your audience?
- What impact will this information have on your target audience?

Tailor need and value statements to appeal to the target audience. Often, the information you include in the need and value pillars goes into the background summary of a study report.

Pillar 4. The Process

Now, let's begin to illustrate the all-encompassing process that goes into designing and evaluating PE analyses and reflect on the art of crafting the experience.

To craft the experience and plan for conducting and evaluating PE analyses, you must be able to visualize your strategy or plan by clearly outlining all "the process" components together. It takes a considerable amount of resources to conduct a thorough and robust evaluation, so understanding the essential parts of "The Process" (or journey) is crucial. You need to understand "**The Process**" and what is needed regardless if you are conducting and evaluating PE analyses. This skill applies to all individual roles.

Chapter 5: Designing and Curating the Experience

There are many moving parts, and The Process to achieve the outcomes is as important as the outcome. The Process is created to illustrate four domains and seven essential elements required to conduct and evaluate PE analyses. It encompasses the addition of items – basically layering on different parts and processes together.

Domains of The Process

You will need to initially outline and assess four domains and then keep the domains in mind throughout the process.

The four major domains include:
- A. Environment
- B. Time
- C. Study Components
- D. The Team

You will need to identify and list what you need in terms of team members, study components, environment, and time initially and likely throughout the whole process.

A. **Environment**

As part of the planning process, identify the infrastructure and the resources around you. Evaluate what is available to you, given what you are trying to answer or achieve. The key is to identify the breadth of the resources you need – or how "sophisticated" you need the resources. It is also critical to understand the institutional barriers and facilitators you will face.

Answer the following questions about the Environment:
- Do you want to conduct CEAs in-house? If so, does your institution have the necessary infrastructure to conduct CEA? The resources you need can depend on if you are performing, evaluating (reviewing) a PE analysis, or implementing a decision from PE analyses.
- What resources are available to you to make this happen?
- What do you have access to at your institution or in your network?
- If you want to implement a new service – do you have the environment, space, etc.? Is this possible?
- Based on your institution and the role you play (designer, doer, or user) – can your institution accommodate what is required for your role?
- Are there any barriers and enablers in your environment for conducting and evaluating PE analyses or implementing recommendations based on PE analyses? It is critical to recognize the limitations of your environment.
- The overarching question to answer is: what are the institutional realities?

Your responses to these questions can change throughout the process.

B. Time

For appropriate scheduling and time management, answer the following questions:
- What is your time frame?
- How quickly do you need the information? How fast do you need to make a decision? The level of detail of your analysis and review may depend on the time you have.
- When do you need to complete the analysis or analysis review?

Answering these questions will assist you with the following items:
- Setting a schedule and agenda
- Creating a timeline for all the elements of The Process like:
  - Setting a deadline for completion of analysis or review.
  - Setting a date for decision-making after completion.

Consider setting dates and reverse engineering everything that needs to get done.

C. Study Components – the Actual Analysis

This domain is where you choose the right analysis to conduct. Consider using the PE Canvas for this domain. The PE Canvas is introduced in Chapter 7.

D. Team

The team is the "staff" or members associated with conducting and evaluating the analysis. The perspectives embedded in The Process come from those who are part of the team or are helping to build or evaluate the analysis. Refer to Chapter 6 for more information on this topic. Make sure to include the strategy you crafted into The Process.

Elements of The Process

There are **seven critical elements** of **The Process** to conduct and evaluate PE analyses. These seven elements are part of both the **PE Lifecycle** and part of **The Process** and play an essential role in the overall analysis course. While it is necessary to plan, be sure to leave room for innovation. Ideas may come up, and there may be instances where you will need to improvise and potentially pivot from your original strategy.

Seven Critical Elements of The Process

1. Defining standards
2. Organization
3. Designing and re-designing
4. Execution or implementation
5. Evaluation or assessment
6. Communication strategies
7. Implementation strategies and processes after completion

1. Defining standards

Define your standards. Set specific, measurable, metric-driven goals and make them relevant to your target audience. Do not forget that you must address both the need and value. This is essential to deliver on what is important to the audience and tailor it to their perspective. The perspective is half the battle. This is where you determine the team's inclusion criteria and exclusion criteria, PE Canvas items, and the resources required.

Use the **"Need"** and **"Value"** Pillars – to answer the following questions:
- What are the critical questions you want to explore? This is an essential and fundamental question when doing research.
- What are you trying to do?
- How are you measuring or defining the "success" of the process? What are your measures of "success," and when would this be considered "complete"? Prioritize success – so what does that mean to you? Consider using the PE Canvas to assist in identifying items to complete.
- What are the outputs of this process? What will it inform? Will you propose a new idea, introduce a new product, or revise existing services or interventions? What will you do after this study is over or after evaluating the analysis or reading it?

Chapter 5: Designing and Curating the Experience

2. Organization

Be organized and create a systematic, structured process for everything you do. In an orderly fashion, work with your team to decide how you will measure progress and prioritize work. Set milestones and leverage benchmarks. Consider creating one or more of the following: a list of routines, a flow chart, item rankings based on priority, or a milestone tracker to assist with organizing, prioritizing, and tracking progress. Be organized and adaptable.

3. Design and Re-Designing

The designing and re-designing element helps you identify any critical problems, solutions, and metrics early and throughout the process. Part of the design process is to continuously reexamination the various plans – which allows for an immediate response. What often happens is that you will **reiterate the design** based on data gathering and learning. Therefore, accept that your plan may change. We continuously adapt and reform what we do to more accurately reflect the realities on the ground. Identify critical issues and elements early on and pivot as needed. Always adjust accordingly based on what you have learned throughout the whole process. You will be designing and re-designing both your teams and your analysis.

- To design your teams, refer to Chapter 6.
- To design your analysis – refer to Chapter 7 for the PE Canvas. Consider using the PE Canvas to build the design of the analysis and understand the basic components of PE analyses.

This book helps you decide what to include or exclude in the designing (and re-designing process). You must always document and be able to explain your rationale when you decide on anything.

4. Execution or Implementation

You need to understand your execution and implementation process to conduct and review a PE analysis before getting started. This helps you find ways to improve the execution, in general.

Impact on Workflow Processes

Map out workflow processes that are required for the execution or evaluation of the analysis. Distinguish all the components that go into executing a PE analysis, emphasizing all four domains: environment, time, study components, and the team.

It would be best to acknowledge that the execution and implementation element might impact workflow processes and workforce time. For example, if this will introduce a new medication or new services, is there is an operational and administrative side to this that will need to be tested? It is crucial to evaluate the workflow processes (especially the operations) and the impact "The Process" will have on workflow.

Continuously reexamine any plans during execution to allow for an immediate response. It would help if you consistently thought about what comes next in The Process during implementation. Do not forget to develop a method to double-check your work.

Data Collection

Develop a data collection and analysis plan (see Chapter 7 for some suggestions). Consider building the data collection process into workflows. Potentially create "shifts" in their workflows, making it easier for individuals to incorporate set metrics and measurable targets for data collection. Create your system or process to track and document data to determine whether you are achieving the desired outcome(s). You will have to clearly articulate where you are getting the data. The PE Canvas may assist here (see Chapter 7). Collect the relevant data and outcomes to make actionable insight from the data.

Increased technology has enabled greater data collection capabilities. Depending on the scope of the analysis and your role, you may consider working with the informatics teams to build systems within electronic health records (EHR) or electronic medical records (EMR) to track desired outcomes.

5. <u>Evaluation or Assessment</u>

Conduct an initial assessment of how all other elements in the process are working to determine actual performance or results. Evaluate any "critical factors" within the team, analysis components, environment, and the timeline to identify challenges and opportunities for improvement. Identify what is going well, what is not working, and what you want to improve. What are the current strengths and weaknesses? Identify any opportunities or challenges you are facing or may anticipate. Many assumptions are made in PE analyses, thus create a system for testing these throughout the process. Be immensely critical of all components of the analysis and interpret the results with caution.

6. <u>Communication Strategies</u>

Once you complete the analysis, decide what you will do with the information. Identify how you want to showcase your work and the ways you want to present your data.

Identify and determine:
- How you will deliver or communicate the information. Numerous options are available, including in the form of a presentation, memo, article, peer-reviewed publication, or maybe an internal-only document. If you know how you will be communicating this information – be sure to prepare ahead of time.
- Whether the communication will be verbal or written.
- Whether it is for internal use only or can it be shared externally. Is it an analysis of internal data that cannot be shared externally? If it can be shared externally, who else will benefit from this information? Can you repeat the analysis across institutions? If you want it presented or published, you will need to check if any institutional review board (IRB) approval is required.

Recognize that you will likely have to communicate these findings to those in different disciplines. Hence, the plan should account for ways to communicate with individuals with diverse backgrounds. Consider communicating results to a broader audience to share and create best practices.

The **six things** you should focus on when **communicating**:
1. Audience
2. Time
3. Content
4. Value
5. Delivery and Style
6. Storytelling – as needed

Start by answering all the questions for each item.

Audience

Know as much about the audience as possible. The more you know about the audience, the better you will tailor the communication – or message(s) to that audience. Consider answering the following:
- Who is the audience? Employees? C-suite? Public? Your immediate team? Is it a team you have not worked with in the past?
- What is your audience's industry? How does it compare to your sector or setting? What are the similarities and differences?
- What is important to them?
- Perspective matters – what are they "seeing"?
- The concept of power in the room: consider the rank and position of the individuals. What influence do these individuals have? What do you anticipate they will do with the information you provide? What do you want them to do with the information? Is what you are stating clear enough for those individuals?

Time

Time helps assess interest, attention span, and attitudes towards the information. Time of the year, month, and day all may impact the data's acceptance and retention. Consider answering the following:
- What else is happening in the setting around this topic? Is there "noise" around the issue you are talking about – e.g., in the news?
- When are you giving the talk, meeting, communication? First thing in the morning? Before or after lunch? End of the day? Their attention is going to vary depending on the time of day.
- Is it during an organizational change? Consider the time within the institution.

Content

Content should reflect the available information and what is still unknown. Content must also reflect the needs of the audience. Communicate both research and real-life experiences. Consider answering the following:
- Are you communicating opinions or evidence-based facts?
- Do you recognize what biases are apparent in the delivery and content development?

Although this may seem that communicating this information is a mix of storytelling and facts or research – the core should still be facts-driven. The specific content items and how you relay those facts depend on the audience.

Value

When people do not see value in something, their attention span shifts elsewhere. Have something worth sharing with a clear call to action and or recommendation(s). Tell them exactly what to do with this information and how it may benefit them.
Consider answering the following:
- Does your communication style and content clearly deliver a benefit to them?
- What do they seek to gain by listening to you or working with you?

Delivery and Style

You will need to determine the mode and style of content delivery.
Consider answering the following:
- What is the mode(s) or format of the delivery of the information? Will it take the form of a research paper, podium or presentation, online summary, etc.? Everything has an appropriate time and place. You do not have to do it all.
- From who's perspective are you delivering the message? Is this the best format to provide the information to this audience?
- Keep in mind any language barriers or cultural differences that may be present.
- If it is in a presentation format, watch your body language. There is a whole science around body language. I recommend seeking additional resources for more information.

Storytelling – as needed

There is power in storytelling. Nevertheless, like every other area, it only works when it is appropriate. If you have only a short time or word length limitations to deliver the specific message or action item, then telling a story, maybe not be the best approach or even appropriate given the format of communication.

7. <u>Implementation Strategies and Process after Completion</u>

Once the PE analysis or review is complete and recommendations are generated, then what? Decide how or if you will use the information generated from this analysis. Consider answering the following:

- Will I make a decision based on the recommendation(s)?
- What will happen if I do take this action or make this decision? What will happen if I do not?
- Will the recommendations result in a work-flow process redesign?

If you have chosen between competing interventions, you now have to set up the transformative processes to implement the intervention chosen. Develop an individualized toolkit for the implementation of the recommendations to your institution.

If you do not have the capabilities to act on the decision rule – is it worth the cost to conduct the study or analysis? **This is a vital question!** You may consider not conducting a study but may consider evaluating one instead. This is often the dilemma between doing your own (and all the resources it entails) vs. assessing a study. But remember, a major limitation or drawback to only evaluating a study is the question of its generalizability to your population of interest.

Up Next

In this chapter, we discussed designing and curating the experience by reviewing the lifecycle of a PE analysis, PE base, and the domains and elements of The Process. In the next chapter, we will discuss building the team for conducting and evaluating PE analyses. This includes the team types, team archetypes, characteristics of the team members, recruiting team members, and designing the team experiences.

CHAPTER 6: BUILDING THE TEAM

Now, let's shift to the team and the skills required to conduct and evaluate pharmacoeconomics (PE) analyses. The importance of teams goes without saying. A fundamental element of building a great product or service is to create a great team. Just as you would create a team before building or incorporating a product or service, the same applies to build a great team to conduct this type of research (or research in general). Effective teams bring shared goals and diverse knowledge to the table. Overall, scaling innovative and impactful interventions requires effective teams.

Outcomes Research (OR) and PE analyses require a considerable amount of resources to perform and one paramount resource being the personnel conducting the studies. It relies on obtaining information from several sources and involves input from numerous individuals. The assortment of data and people (those who will collect, assess, and decide) are all interconnected and influence an analysis output.

The questions we ask and the problems we are trying to address are multifaceted; therefore, our teams should be too. The experiences and skill set of the individuals and teams involved in assessing value must also be multidimensional since value itself is complex. Our problems were not created by one factor, and therefore our solutions should not be evaluated by only one lens. Step back and think of better ways to objectively create the teams we need to conduct and assess PE analyses.

This section aims to answer the common questions individuals have concerning teams in PE analyses. These questions include:
- How do you go about setting up your team?
- Whom do you bring on board?
- What skills do you need to perform a PE analysis?

Use design thinking when creating your teams.

When building your team, you should focus on growth-oriented leadership – one that utilizes design thinking. This helps to create teams that will work towards something bigger, scalable, and more sustainable. One of your goals may be to increase the presence of PE at institutions. A suggestion for any institution looking to partake in creating an innovative strategy is to create portfolios of the future, including creating individual portfolios, team portfolios, and intervention portfolios.

Team Types

Build Your Team Out

Be creative in how you build your team. Building your team is innovation in itself and often comes from and with artistic collaborations and by effectively mobilizing resources. Gather in the most appropriate – or "right" – professionals to create your teams to help identify all the relevant components and inputs of the analysis. The team members are vital to identifying and formulating the question, methods, analysis, and utilization of the information generated from these analyses. The team collectively develops these items throughout the process.

Consider creating <u>two main types</u> of teams at your institution or group: PE Conduct Team and the PE Evaluate Team.

PE Conduct Team

The team that **conducts** the analysis. If you are interested in doing a PE analysis, consider creating a PE Conduct Team. This team **conducts, executes, or performs** the PE analysis. Members of this team will also have the skillset to assess PE studies and thus can be used to assist in the evaluation of PE studies. They may also serve as expert consultants to those internally seeking to evaluate PE studies.

PE Evaluate Team

The team that **evaluates** the analysis. If your institution or group does not plan to conduct PE analyses, a team can be formed to assess relevant PE analyses as they emerge to determine whether they may be considered part of the decision-making process. Evaluation of a PE analysis can be an individual effort (as it is often done) but may also require more than one person for consideration into broader, macro-level decision-making. The team could potentially be part of the Pharmacy & Therapeutics (P&T) committee, or P&T members may be part of the PE Evaluation team.

If you are seriously considering incorporating PE analyses into your decision-making process, consider creating a **PE Helpline,** which includes a database of individuals with experience performing and evaluating OR or PE to serve as a resource when decision questions arise. Drug information specialists act in this role at many institutions and health systems.

Here are a few recommendations:
- Identify who in your institution has done similar work (or has the skill sets required) and use them as an expert resource in conducting or evaluating PE studies.
- If your institution already has a PE Conduct Team, consider using them as a resource for evaluating PE analyses. Seek out these individuals to add them to the team. Have them either be a part of the PE Evaluate Team or part of the PE Helpline.
- Use various frameworks (similar to those in this chapter and the PE Canvas in Chapter 7) and resources to help identify individuals for your teams.
- Consider continuously building your skill sets to conduct or evaluate PE analyses by using tools (such as this book) that assist you in identifying the various elements, best practices, and skills needed for both conducting and evaluating PE analyses.

The Core Team

Be thoughtful and intentional in your team design and whom you allow on your team. Distinguish what each team member brings to the table in terms of skills and potential contribution. Clearly articulate what you expect of each member and where you would like them to be most involved.

Begin with answering the questions:
- Who is good to have on your team?
- Who do you bring on board?
- Evaluate and ask, "Are the right people part of the team"? It is essential to identify the "right" people early. You may likely come back to this question as things change throughout the process.

The core team discussed below is the team conducting PE analyses. You do not need all these individuals to evaluate PE analyses, but it would be insightful to get these individuals' perspectives. The individuals you have as part of the core team will help build the relevant information and efficiently disseminate it to your target audience. Blend professionals from other departments and practitioners from industry settings and practices into the team to create more diverse teams with insightful perspectives.

Cross the borders of different disciplines and break the silos within silos. You can either recruit them as members of the team or as experts. It would be best to differentiate between the individuals who are "actively doing" the work in the analyses versus those that are part of the conversation to build, edit, and make the model relevant. Make sure that those in the conversation can be part of the conversation. Include all the relevant stakeholders, at least in the discussions – to seek the right perspective.

It is ideal to have those <u>who create the innovation</u> and <u>those who use it</u> in one team – or at the very least, communicating. For an intervention to fulfill its "value" capacity, you want the communication between those who create the innovation and those who use it to be strong. If you desire the impact of your analysis to extend beyond a team or institution, consider welcoming individuals from the "outside" into the conversations.

Team Archetypes

The Team Archetype is the "perfect" example of a group of individuals with the skills and background that a PE analysis may require and are therefore essential to have on the team. It is central to pay close attention to the individuals' diverse experiences conducting or evaluating PE analyses to ensure that all the facets of these analyses are covered. Studies that incorporate various backgrounds and perspectives may be deemed more "realistic" as they may better reflect realities on the ground.

It does not mean that you cannot do a PE analysis if you do not have all these skills. It just means that you may be leveraging the particular expertise or "Type" or "Focus Area" of that individual at some point in the process. Consider either having a specific person with that background or a person with a background that covers multiple skills. Either have the person or the skills this person provides.

You will find yourself blending individuals with various expertise areas for the team. The diverse collection of team members can better assist with highlighting the relevant information in the various elements of the process. As previously noted, idea synthesis from multiple disciplines is required; therefore, crafting the right team will notably support the process.

The potential team members are differentiated by "Types" or "Focus Areas" below – basically, by areas of specialization, domains of expertise, position, or background.

Team Archetype: The 10 Focus Areas or Types

1. Healthcare provider or individual with a clinical background
2. Researcher with experience in outcomes and health service research
3. Statistician or analyst
4. Health economist
5. Drug information specialist
6. Decision-maker(s)
7. Partners or collaborators
8. Advisory board of experts: internal and external advisory boards
9. Patient advocates
10. Mentors

Details of the ten are below:

<u>Healthcare Provider or Individual with a Clinical Background</u>

These are the individuals providing the clinical service (e.g., visits, procedures) and/or prescribing, dispensing, or administering the medications. Examples of individuals that are part of this type include physicians (MDs or DOs), pharmacist (RPh or PharmD), dentist (DDS, DMD), physician assistant (PA), physical therapist (PT), nurse (RN), Nurse Practitioners (NP), and Advanced Practice Nurses (APN).

These individuals are part of the process of delivering the product or service. They understand how to clinically manage patients and understand the impact of the interventions in practice. These individuals may also have added credentials, expertise, or training in PE and OR (e.g., received a master's in this area or completed a fellowship) and would be considered someone with multiple domains of expertise.

<u>Researcher with Experience in Outcomes and Health Service Research</u>

Researchers with backgrounds and expertise in OR, such as health service researchers or epidemiologists, are the next type. These individuals have eclectic skills that can be applied to several diverse questions and specialties. These individuals may overlap in skills or experiences of another "type."

<u>Statistician or Analyst</u>

PE is very statistics-rich and data-dense; therefore, you need someone who can understand the statistical methodology to choose sound statistical methods and analyze the data appropriately. This helps avoid making recommendations based on improper or weak analyses.

<u>Health Economist</u>

Costs are a central pillar in PE analyses. An individual with a background in economics (especially health economics) would contribute to evaluating appropriate cost methodology to determine relevant cost inputs and assess the economic impact of an intervention.

Drug Information Specialist

Members of the drug information services team are trained in and involved in several relevant activities, such as:[25,106]
- providing literature evaluation and drug information
- developing and disseminating medication-use policies
- participating in health outcomes initiatives
- coordinating formulary management initiatives
- working with the pharmacy informatics teams and systems.

These individuals have experience communicating interventions and recommendations within their institutions – to decision-makers, providers, and even patients – in various forms and across healthcare systems.

Decision-Maker(s)

These are the individuals that may use the information generated from the PE analyses to make a decision. Identify the decision-makers that will likely use this information, as this will allow you to tailor your message better to meet those decision-makers' specific concerns and needs. Are they in the public sector, the healthcare sector, patient or caregiver, or family (among many others)? Make sure all the relevant perspectives are incorporated. See Chapter 1 for a summary of the various decision-makers.

Partners or Collaborators

Partners and collaborators can offer needed resources and add perspectives to the process that may be valuable to your analysis.

Advisory Board of Experts

Consider seeking advice from people outside of your team by creating subset teams or advisory boards. As you design your study or try to understand the actual realities on the ground, look for individuals on the ground to gain insight from the frontlines. Since the perspective considerably influences PE, make sure you incorporate feedback and guidance from relevant internal and external stakeholders.

Look for individuals on the ground who will likely be affected by the decision and any content experts pertinent to the question at hand. Ultimately, you want them to fill an information gap to answer the decision question sufficiently.

Answer the following questions:
- Who are the pertinent experts, individuals on the ground, specific organizations, or institutions?
- From whom will you seek advice?

Approach experts for greater insight on the topic, as the decision will likely affect them. Look for experts involved in the practice since they will speak to what is done in the "real world."
- Seek out people who are well versed in the industry and understand the factors according to their influence over the problem at hand.
- Recognize what advice these individuals are unable to provide and seek out other advisors who can.
- Identify who the intervention(s) impacts and then figure out the best way to incorporate them into the building process.
- Discover who is currently solving this problem or working to solve this problem both internally and externally.

This approach enables those on the ground to take some ownership of and participate in identifying the most relevant solution.

To understand some of the challenges: 1) ask those on the front line to walk you through it., 2) organize and participate in a "listening tour" with these individuals, and 3) identify what questions you need to answer as a result. This will also help you identify new needs for the use of the information. These experts can also be individuals with expertise in the various Team Archetype Focus Areas.

The expert(s) you choose may also depend on how wide of a net you want to cast, the decision context, and the research question.

For example, you can choose from a variety of experts, including industry experts (pharmaceutical companies, pharmacy benefit management companies, managed care organizations, other health systems), academicians, political analysts, policy experts, and social scientists.

If the intervention is related to a specific disease state or specialty (e.g., cardiology, infectious disease), make sure someone from that care team is either a team member or an external expert.

Internal Advisory Boards

Internal advisory board members are those within your institution. You may consider adding them to the team or at least connecting with them as experts to consult throughout the process.

To find internal experts, answer the following questions:
- What professionals (within the institution) will be impacted by the question or problem or potential solution?
- Who is impacted both in terms of processes and outcomes?

External Advisory Boards

External advisory board members are individuals outside of your institution. The questions we are asking and working to address often go beyond the boundaries of our institutions. If you are not in the setting with which the question is applicable, it is recommended that you seek external experts in practice. For example, if you are in an academic setting, and a relevant or affected institution is off-campus, seek outside experts within the appropriate environment.

Patient Advocates

Depending on the project's scope or analysis, you may consider adding consumer representatives or members of national organizations or patient advocacy groups whose work is to advocate for and speak to the realities of specific patient populations.[40] These individuals can also be a part of your advisory group and not the actual team members. If you do not take this approach, find a way to make sure that patient preferences are included.

Chapter 6: Building the Team

<u>Mentors</u>

Behind the scenes, consider having formal or informal mentors who will help you or your team successfully complete and adopt the analysis.

In summary, the main focus groups include **teams**, **decision-makers**, **partners/ collaborators**, **experts**, and **mentors**.

Characteristics of the Team Members

The world of PE analyses consists of a diverse collection of researchers, clinicians, decision-makers, patient advocates, and researchers working together. All these individuals help reflect the realities on the ground and individuals involved in delivering care. The information generated from these types of analyses may be of interest to all.

As you are building your team, there are **four main characteristics** you should look for in team members. These include:
1. Have the skills needed
2. Diverse in terms of experiences, skill sets, and perspectives
3. Collaborative
4. Nonconventional thinkers

1. Have the skills needed

Match individuals with the skills and expertise required. These are the skills you've identified before seeking out team members. Because of the breadth of knowledge required, taking the time to make sure you have the skills needed will assist in overcoming any technical obstacles experienced during the process. The ability to communicate the results and recommendations to those that use it (users) can influence its uptake. Overall, identify what skills each member brings to the table, leverage the individual's strengths, and divide work to match skills accordingly.

Core Skills

Now, you need to determine the skills you need to equip yourself and your team to conduct and evaluate PE analyses. Create your bucket list of skills by leveraging the skills list below. Let's start with the "Must-Haves" skills and then review the "Added Benefit" skills.

"Must-Haves" Skills

These are skills that team members need to conduct and/or evaluate PE analyses effectively. Some overarching transferable skills across disciplines include:
- Retrieval of evidence
- Identifying applicable metrics
- Data collection
- Statistics and data analysis

- Attention to detail
- Communication skills – both written and verbal.

Skills more pertinent to PE analyses include:
- *Technical knowledge* in their designated field or domain is critical – whether it is in economic, clinical, or humanistic outcomes or health outcomes research in general. The technical limitations of the team members often threaten the quality, viability, and applicability of PE analyses. One must have a background and understanding of the appropriate methodology associated with OR and PE analyses.
- *Clinical background* is essential since these are healthcare-specific questions. One needs to have the clinical on the ground experience to translate and apply it to real-world practice.

"Added Benefit" Skills

These skills include those that extend beyond the "must-have" skills and eventually add to the process, either in content or efficiency. An example of an "added benefit" is extensive previous history conducting this type of research, which may positively influence the quality of the analysis and speed at which it is completed.

Try to avoid redundancies of expertise (adding similar experts or focus areas) unless those individuals add something unique to the team. There is no need to have four clinical pharmacists who are doing the same thing unless they are unique somehow. For example, they may serve different populations of interest, have additional skills sets in methodology, or offer a unique perspective or domain of expertise.

2. **Diversity of experiences, skill sets, and perspectives**

There are positive ripple effects for working with others from different disciplines. The best teams are those with diverse skill sets and views. Diversity permits for divergent thoughts – it enables people to think differently – and ignites creativity. Diversity sparks exciting discussions and adds context, expertise, and foresight to make the time spent and the outcomes more meaningful. Team members with diverse backgrounds assist in developing curated messages to communicate to targeted, relevant audiences and a wide variety of users.

The ability to conduct this research and work with professions from various backgrounds will increase your reach and ability to continue demonstrating your value across healthcare and beyond. When diverse individuals are on your research teams, they become more aware of the impact you make – even if they are not doing the clinical work. One's web of influence substantially grows with more participation and insight from key stakeholders who influence – and are influenced by – the decision question at hand and benefit from realistic solutions. How we take care of our patients in healthcare (as part of a diverse team) is how we should design our projects. Our patients are cared for by a group of assorted professionals (each adds value in some way), and our project teams should reflect this as well. Our professionals, teams, and projects should add value to patients and the intended population(s). We should utilize expertise in various disciplines to find innovative, collaborative solutions.

To effectively build solutions, have various perspectives in your conversations. Ideas for tackling issues and methods to solve these problems grow exponentially with diverse perspectives. If a team is chosen well, they will welcome contrasting opinions and views as examples of various realities on the ground. This is especially relevant if the issues at hand are complex and multidimensional – which they usually are in healthcare. Make sure that diversity of thought and perspectives is present within the team. You want dynamic people who bring new perspectives to ensure the success of the analysis.

The strength of a team is in the skills and perspectives each provides. Seek new ways to partner with diverse professionals, and do not forget to use design thinking.

3. Collaborative

It is essential to build collaborative teams. A team should collaborate in a way that leverages the experiences of each team member. A collaborative team works to continuously streamline and integrate the differences in skill sets and perspectives throughout the process. This skill will prove to be especially important as you bring in experts and seek out opinions.

4. Nonconventional thinkers

Teams should not only include those with technical expertise but also include non-conventional thinkers. Seek out and work with those who think "out of the box" to question conventional approaches and find suitable solutions.

The Team's Influence in Decision-Making

A key question to answer as you are forming your team is, **does anyone in your team influence decision-making?** Do not just focus on having a diverse team but rather identify what power and influence they have in doing something with the outcome of the analysis. Strive to have someone with influence as a part of your team.

For each team member, answer the following questions:
- What is their perspective?
- What are his or her contributions to the team and beyond the project?
- Do they influence decision-making?
- What power do they have, and to whom?
- What do you want them to do with that power?

Carefully craft a list of individuals who need to be on the team table – that is, those that can help steer the analysis or recommendations – versus those that may only want to know (a "nice to know") the information generated from the team. Determine whether you will benefit from having the individual as part of the team or someone you would like for the background.

Recruiting Team Members

Now to recruit the team members, follow the steps outlined below.

Steps to Recruiting Team Members

1. Identify the skills required to enlist the necessary team members. Use the Skills and Focus Areas outlined before to recruit. Since you know what you need, you can actively recruit team members. Recognize each member's limitations and seek out advice from those who will fill those gaps.
2. Evaluate where you are "located." Assess your environment and inquire about what personnel is available to you (both on the department and organizational level). For example, those in academia have an opportunity to collaborate with individuals across departments and colleges.
3. Determine how much you want to or can recruit internally versus externally.
    a. <u>Internally</u>: Understand what potential sources of talent are available to you at your location. It is not about finding the smartest people you can find – it is about finding smart people to perform the skills you need.
    b. <u>Externally</u>: Assess how much external assistance you need. The extent you can recruit externally for a specific project depends on your institution. Therefore, check with your institution to see what rules apply. It is important to recognize when to add to the team and when to seek advice – e.g., you may not always need external consultants on the team. This can depend on your setting and what resources you have available.
4. Identify and leverage partnerships. Pick partners to advance your initiatives. Make a list of your current partners and assess whether you need to build on or improve your connections. Among your list of actual and potential partners, recognize who you need to partner with to accomplish your goals. Be sure to set a timeline for collaboration.
5. Recruit diverse, collaborative team members.

Team Assessments

Assess the "health" of the team by mapping out the contributions of each member to evaluate further what is missing. Conducting team assessments helps identify gaps in knowledge among the team at the beginning and throughout the process. It also aids in identifying any barriers or obstacles to the completion of activities. Each team member is expected to be honest and transparent about their limitations to fill the gaps adequately.

During the initial team assessment and throughout the process:

1. Identify the skills and activities needed.
2. Clearly define what skills each team member brings individually compared to their skills and contribution to a team. Identify whether any of the individual skills work in synergy with the other team members. This allows you to understand each team member's background and what skills they have to leverage.
3. Assign activities to perform based on identified skills (self and group) and backgrounds of interest. Avoid merely assigning a task, but rather have each team member commit to the job.
4. Set expectations of each team member to know what is required of them and then affix a deadline for each activity.
5. Create a system to edit the information inputted in the team assessments and include a transparent process for team member evaluations throughout the process.

Consider creating a tracking system with a table similar to Table 1 for the team assessments. You do not have to use this table exactly how it is presented. You can create your own table and include the items you believe would be most beneficial for a team assessment.

Table 1: Team Assessments Tracking System

Skills Needed	List Items
Activities Needed *Use the Pharmacoeconomics Canvas to make a list of activities required based on the type of analysis and methodology you will use.*	
Individual *Name & title*	
Skills Present *Consider breaking it down to "must-have" and "added benefit."*	
Activities to Perform *What will they provide?* *Identify critical activities they will conduct. Activities can vary based on what needs to be done.*	
Deadline(s) *Add a deadline or milestone to each item.*	

Designing the Team Experience

The Lead Designer

The first step to designing the team experience is to designate a "leader" or what is often called the "project manager" or the "primary investigator." In our case, we will call him/her the Lead Designer. This individual will take ownership, lead the project management efforts, and oversee the organization of all the pieces.

Step 1 of Designing the Team Experience

Define a point person or the Lead Designer.

Primary role and functions of the Lead Designer include:

- Works with team members to develop the research agenda and organize meetings.
- Ensures suitable communication strategies among team members.
- Develops the process plan based on actionable items.
- Recaps the research question throughout the process.
- Works with the team to outline what needs to be done and creates a list of all the activities to be performed.
- Delegates responsibilities and tasks to team members as needed.
- Holds the master spreadsheet (or whatever method is used for tracking), summarizing all activities to be performed by each member.
- Establishes and maintains accordance with deadlines and holds team members accountable.
- Actively engages team members based on their needs and progress.
- Engages external stakeholders as needed. Stakeholders can include those with a shared interest in the analysis.

Design Meetings

As for the meetings, "Team Meetings" have been renamed here to "Design Meetings." The lead designer steers design meetings; however, they are crafted with input in collaboration with everyone on the team. To make the most of your design meetings, below are a few suggestions the team should do during the first meeting and revisit for each meeting.

Team Tasks Meeting

1. Be organized and stick to a schedule.
2. Establish principles or ground rules for the meeting.
3. Discuss communication styles.
4. Form goals.
5. Create an action plan for each element and assign a person to that item.
6. Discuss the documentation process.
7. Discuss the internal and external use of information.
8. Discuss expectations for the next meeting.
9. Evaluate the quality of the meetings.

Let's discuss each in more detail:

1. Be organized and stick to a schedule

Follow an agenda with clearly defined expectations. It may be created pre-meeting or collectively during the first five minutes of a meeting. Dedicate time to identify and establish metrics, milestones, benchmarks to success. Set a detailed timeline and establish deadlines. Consider taking meeting minutes, if helpful, and consider delegating it to a specific or different team member each time. Always ask someone to write things down. Consider pre-scheduling consistent weekly meetings in advance, at least once a week, meeting – similar to the concept of team huddles. This approach promotes collaborative learning.

2. Establish principles or ground rules for meetings

Communicate the principles or ground rules for the meetings early and often – and continuously review them in subsequent sessions. These are not meant to be restrictive but rather act to help facilitate more efficient meetings. Determine the team's decision-making process. Map out the decision-making process for each team member's deliverable

Chapter 6: Building the Team

throughout the process to determine how the information is shared and what makes it go to the "next level" in the process. Create a method for shared decision-making by first identifying how you want to proceed with this approach. Consider defining shared decision-making individually and then collectively as a team.

3. <u>Discuss communication styles</u>

Create a deliberate process for working together – including individual communication preferences and styles. Due to differences in preferences, be sure to reach a consensus on what communication style will be used moving forward. To create more efficient knowledge sharing sessions – be clear on communication styles and best modes of collaboration. Continuously evaluate and experiment with new methods of teamwork. Seek new ways to communicate with diverse professionals – especially early on in the process.

4. <u>Form goals</u>

Understand all the elements of your agenda and form your collective goals. Create a vision highlighting anticipated team member contributions, and be sure to establish a clear direction for where you are going. Design how your collaborations will work and foster unconventional thinking. Determine a system for member accountability.

5. <u>Create an action plan for each element of the process and assign a person to that item</u>

Set realistic expectations of team members and concrete steps moving forward. Write down your action steps. Assign areas of expertise and delegate. Delegation is essential with all the moving parts. Design your plan keeping in mind how you will delegate. Deadlines and tasks should be frequently assessed. Depending on how large the group gets, consider small groups to review concepts or results. Fill out team assessment to assign tasks or activities. Duties may fluctuate – anticipate this and adjust accordingly. You may consider having each member fill out their own skill table before creating the team master document.

6. <u>Discuss the documentation process</u>

This entails how the information will be collected, shared, or used – both internally and externally. Here you are focusing on how you "document the science."

7. <u>Discuss the internal and external use of information</u>

Determine how the information will be presented before and during the meeting. For example, the agenda with the assigned tasks to be completed by each person should be sent out a few days before the meeting to ensure review from team members. During the meeting, each should come prepared and know who will report out and what is required. Identifying how you will use the information generated through your analysis can help determine the communication style used from the beginning and help you determine what documentation may be needed. This assists in reevaluating and reiterating how this information will be used – internally vs. externally or both.

8. <u>Discuss expectations for the next meeting</u>

Set clear expectations for current and future meetings. Assumptions are problematic if not spelled out. Remember, meetings should focus on outputs and meeting metrics identified.

9. <u>Evaluate the quality of the meetings</u>

Create a system to reflect on your processes in the meetings. As you build the needs of the project, recognize that needs may change. Always check, verify, and adapt your encounters to maximize efficiency and impact. Use meeting time to recap progress and any additional items pending. Incorporate a reflective component of your developments in the meeting. Have the team evaluate how well the strategies are working for the team members. Assess the quality of the meetings themselves and the achievements produced early and frequently. Continuously reexamine your proposed plan, as this allows for an immediate response. Consider creating a scorecard (or report card) of how you track progress. This may assist you in determining what is working and what is not. The results produced by your time as a team – both collaborating and producing – is what counts. The outputs should be the essential core of the meetings.

Create your Own Team Culture

No matter how small a team is, a sound and positive team culture should exist. Create a data-driven, positive, patient-centric team culture from the beginning to create momentum for the remaining time together. This is critical early on in the recruiting stage. The team culture must be responsive, inclusive, and quickly able to adapt to change. The culture should be dedicated to openness to learn from each other. Nurture innovative spirit in all the team members. Teams should consider themselves mini-innovation groups.

Create a culture where help-seeking is the norm. All individuals should value team camaraderie and trust. Make it easier for people to ask for help. Humility is also vital in teams. Acknowledge what you are good at and what you are not. Team members should feel comfortable recognizing their shortcomings and limitations. Try to minimize hierarchy and avoid micromanagement. Have one person (the Lead Designer) for logistical, operational oversight, and identify the decision-making process that involves everyone's input.

As you work on the analysis, build the culture focused on the need and value of PE analyses at your institution. The team will likely face the challenge of creating a suitable environment for this type of work if one does not exist. The value systems and organizational perspective for this type of analysis can facilitate or hinder the process. In some cases, the challenge is not just a knowledge gap; but rather a lack of motivation to conduct or evaluate these types of analyses. Therefore, it is critical to creating a robust internal team culture.

Up Next

In this chapter, we discussed building the team for conducting and evaluating PE analyses. This includes the team types, team archetypes, characteristics of the team members, recruiting team members, and designing the team experiences. In the next chapter, we will review the standards and approaches to conduct and evaluate PE analyses. The PE canvas is introduced and explained in detail, including a statement of its use.

CHAPTER 7: THE PHARMACOECONOMICS CANVAS

Guidance on Pharmacoeconomics Analyses

Although there are no standard guidelines or "standard rules" for conducting and reporting economic analyses, many organizations, researchers, and editors – as well as the economic evaluation community – all still call for a more standardized approach for pharmacoeconomics (PE) analyses.[1,25,26,29,42,44,73,77,87,125,128,139,154,175,176] Many have called for a minimum set of criteria so that essential items may not be overlooked – and allows for criticism of methods and biases during evaluation.[1,26,29,42,44,53,73,77,125,128,139,154,175-177]

There are "acceptable methods"[29] and practice standards available.[1,25,26,29,42,44,73,77,125,139,154,175,176] These methods are summarized in various submissions and reporting guidelines, checklists, and recommendations in the literature. Many of these report minimum criteria. [1,25,26,29,42-44,53,73,77,125,139,154,175-177] Researchers have produced numerous checklists – like the Consolidated Health Economic Evaluation Reporting Standards (CHEERS) – for steps to conduct and evaluate economic analyses.[138,139,154]

Standards have emerged from reputable organizations and researchers to improve the quality and transparency of economic analyses.[1,26,29,42-44,53,73,77,81,86,125,139,154,175-178] Guidelines and recommendations have been created to reduce inconsistencies of methodology and the lack of transparency of these analyses.[28,42,177] Informal and unstructured methods are currently available. The ultimate goal of a standard approach is to help increase quality, consistency, and comparability across studies to support the decision-making process.

To improve the quality of cost-effectiveness analysis (CEA) and allow for comparability, it is suggested to use a standard method – or a reference case. A reference case follows the standard set of methods for analysis, allowing you to compare different studies of the same type, evaluate tradeoffs, and make more informed allocation decisions.[77,98,128]

Many of the "best practices" for economic analyses suggested by various groups recommend similar items, such as greater transparency, higher quality of evidence, long-term impact data on outcomes, and a **"statement of intended use"** – that is, to make it clear how you intend to use this information.[26,42,179-184] Efforts to improve transparency include providing the details of the analyses in an appendix – since the restriction in the length of the articles limit their ability to be fully transparent. Experts have suggested that it is likely that task force recommendations have positively influenced the quality of PE and OR studies.[175]

There are items that reviewers, researchers, and ultimately decision-makers look for in these analyses. These are standards that reviewers of this literature may require when publishing. Journal editors have endorsed the use of such available reporting guidelines.[139] Your work may be criticized based on standards set forth by an organization or journal. Remember, journals will critique your methods based on their requirements; therefore, it is essential to check these before submitting the analysis or manuscript for review. Guidance on the methodology and best practices for economic analyses are frequently modified and continue to evolve. Continuously check for the latest recommendations when conducting or evaluating PE analyses.

Guidelines are particularly helpful if you use economic analyses to inform decision-making. This is one reason countries who use the information generated from these economic analyses to inform their decision have more standardized, agreed-upon guidelines. Nevertheless, even with all this guidance, varying opinions on the best approaches and methods remain.[29] Several items are still debated in guidelines and recommendations and can vary based on the geographical location, institution, specific decision-maker, and the perspectives of the creator and user. The Professional Society for Health Economics and Outcomes Research (ISPOR) is a resource for obtaining guidelines for countries across the globe.[29,185]

Introduction to the Pharmacoeconomics Canvas

How the PE Canvas Came to Fruition

The methods associated with these analyses take a considerable amount of time and resources – hence it is critical to be organized and plan ahead. Agencies have encouraged the development of material to assist with the interpretation and application of PE analyses.[20] It has also been recommended to use a written protocol at the onset to help outline and detail all the necessary components of the analysis.[77,128] Built off the continual need to provide a comprehensive framework and create tools to improve our probability of technical success; the PE Canvas was born.

Summary of Various Elements that Went into Making the Canvas

This book complements the existing resources and integrates several other key elements and processes to getting started with PE analyses. It takes a unique approach by using a macro-level holistic approach to the elements of PE and getting started – including the personnel involved.

The contents and recommendations found in this chapter, and the PE Canvas, are consistent with and incorporate various elements from numerous guidelines, checklists, and researchers' strategies across the major players in PEOR.[1,25,26,29,42-44,53,73,77,112,125,139,154,175,176-184,187] This chapter also integrates several additional items to build a holistic view in an easy to follow, easy to read, visual format.

It integrates the steps, standards, best practices of evidence-based medicine (EBM), PE, decision analysis, systematic review, data collection, checklists, recommendations, and numerous other elements into a canvas to serve as the foundational building blocks. The "blocks" found in the PE Canvas include elements that are generally agreed upon as a minimum set of features or criteria. The specific criteria can vary depending on the type of PE analysis conducted.

The various checklists and strategies are continuously updated; therefore, it is advised that you always check for the latest recommendations as you conduct or evaluate PE analyses.

The Goal of the PE Canvas

The PE Canvas helps you navigate the intricacies of the analysis process. It attempts to simplify the complexity and makes it straight forward enough to integrate it into a practitioner's or decision-makers thought process. It introduces you to the basic terms to help you understand the landscape of PE analysis methodology and application. It highlights the major considerations and assists in identifying the right challenges and proper context. It can be considered an "all-in-one" canvas as it contains elements that go into conducting, reporting, and evaluating in a user-friendly format.

The PE Canvas helps decision-makers make a connection between elements – when both conducting or evaluating these analyses. The PE Canvas gives the researchers and decision-makers autonomy in choosing suitable methods appropriate for the study. Examples of specific approaches are included, yet they are not the only ones available. The canvas gives you the flexibility to choose what methods are best for you and your decision question.

There are several goals to having a canvas. These include:
- Provide an easy roadmap for those that are conducting or evaluating the analyses.
- Provide a structure for which to build during the process.
- Improve our capacity to conduct and evaluate the literature.
- Improve the quality and transparency of PE analyses conducted.

The hope is that it allows the information that is generated to be more useful in practice.

An Approach to Conduct and Evaluate PE Analyses

To start, you have to answer the question:
Will you be conducting or evaluating a PE analysis?

No matter if you are conducting or evaluating a PE analysis, you must know what goes into designing the analysis. Note: "analysis" and "study" may be used interchangeably throughout the book. Whether you create it or just read it, you have to evaluate it. It is critical to move from insight into action. Do not just evaluate it – also recognize how you can use it.

Whether you are conducting or evaluating a PE analysis, you can use the PE Canvas to assess the foundation and components of the analysis. Remember, these analyses are complex. The Canvas will help you identify factors to consider when conducting and evaluating PE research.

If you are **conducting PE analyses**, use the canvas as a tool to get started. It serves as a framework to conduct the work that a PE analysis entails. If you plan on also submitting an analysis as a paper to a specific journal, check the organizations' reporting guidelines for directions before submitting it.

When performing economic analyses, the general process uses the evidence we have to fill in the model, make assumptions, and then account for uncertainty. There are several limitations to the process; therefore, it is crucial to interpret the results with caution.

If you are **evaluating or interpreting a PE analysis**, you will need a process for systematically reviewing the PE literature. The PE Canvas can help to evaluate the analysis and understand the various elements methodically. Due to the nature of these studies, you will be evaluating PE analyses more frequently rather than conducting them.

How to Use the Pharmacoeconomics Canvas

The PE Canvas goes beyond a "step by step" approach and helps you craft the **core** creative concept for PE analyses. It is essential to visualize your strategy – as it is much easier when you can see all the pieces together!

The PE Canvas is a framework or skeleton of the critical components that drive conducting and evaluating PE analyses. A canvas approach is used for simplicity and to help envision and connect all the components. Just as you would use the checklists, guidelines, and recommendations for PE analyses, consider using the PE Canvas to get started.

The PE Canvas has three main frames and includes 22 building blocks.

The PE Canvas uses a "reference case" approach – or a suggested standard method for performing economic analyses. The canvas has the foundational building blocks for a PE analysis and acts as a platform for continuously evaluating the elements of these analyses. It provides an information base that you can utilize to create lists to keep track of things you need to look for, do, and consider. It attempts to break down the analyses into smaller, more manageable components. It also provides order to the foundational skills needed to perform or evaluate this type of work.

The elements in the canvas are not itemized rules but building blocks. The canvas allows room for customization based on your needs and perspectives – recognizing that you will likely keep changing your approach regarding what to include or exclude throughout the process. Researchers are also encouraged to create and choose their own approach based on the basics provided and design what is appropriate for the context and question at hand. That is, discover your own approach based on what you have read and learned within the discipline.

The PE Canvas is meant for decision-makers, students, researchers, and anyone interested in conducting, reporting, and/or evaluating PE analyses. Any professional making healthcare decisions will likely come across these analyses and at least review a PE analysis now or in the future. The canvas acknowledges that decision-makers vary in preferences, needs, authority, influence, and impact of the decision question and context.

Next, **develop an action plan** for all the blocks of the canvas and regularly review it. Look at the big picture and pull the layers back on each block. From there, you can then start to focus on the smaller items. Turn each block into a question to assess whether you or the analysis creators have completed the task. Go through the canvas and ask yourself, for each block, is this item addressed? Assess what was conducted and if it was correctly performed. Consider adding a checkmark by each block once completed.

In other words – answer the following **universal questions for each block**:
- Was this block completed?
- If so, was it done appropriately? Did it include all the necessary elements?
- If not, was that appropriate to exclude?
- Was the rationale for each choice made provided?

The PE Canvas is meant to be used as an additional tool or resource for PE analyses and decision-making. It should not be the only item used to make a decision.

Since cost-effectiveness analysis (CEA) is the standard for measuring value, this canvas highlights the major blocks that go into conducting and evaluating CEAs. All the blocks will apply when comparing interventions with similar non-equivalent outcomes – such as in cases of CEA and cost-utility analysis (CUA). The canvas may be used with different types of PE analyses, although you may find yourself not using each block.

How much weight or priority you give to each block depends on your specific analysis. Like other checklists and guidance, no priority weight is given to each element.[77,128]

Transparency in your methods is imperative. Be transparent about your methods so that others can replicate them and adequately compare the analysis with their institution or situation. This assists the readers in assessing the application of the recommendations. Readers will want to know how to recreate the analysis and whether the decision question and result can help inform decisions at their institution.

Chapter 7: The Pharmacoeconomics Canvas

Statement on Use of the PE Canvas

This book and the PE Canvas are an introduction to the fundamentals and should be used as a resource. It is meant to serve as a roadmap or "state of mind" and not a "rule book." Similar to other recommendations – this canvas is not intended to be prescriptive.[125] Consider this book and the PE canvas, in general, as a reference handbook and not an all-inclusive itemized list. It provides you a list of questions to consider as you embark on getting started with PE analyses. Professionals are encouraged to add it to their resources as they construct their own unique toolkits for the skills they need to acquire for PE analyses.

Consider using the PE Canvas in addition to other decision-making tools or strategies.

Not every analysis will include everything in the canvas, and everything may not be applicable in all decision questions. It is challenging to have one canvas include all relevant items for every decision context due to the differences in perspective, decision questions, and context.[45,125] However, this canvas provides a skeleton to which the decision-makers or researcher can follow and input information accordingly. The PE Canvas allows for this flexibility.

Each block will be discussed very briefly. It is meant to tell you what you need to know – or what to learn more about – not be the resource for everything you need to know.

As the discipline grows and more of these analyses are conducted, the details of the recommendations will continuously be updated and refined.[25]

Carefully critique PE analyses and interpret the results with caution.

When publishing this type of research in peer-reviewed journals, it is recommended that you consult the journal for reporting guidelines, criteria for inclusion of items, and methodology requirements before submitting it. Consider using the PE Canvas during journal club (or article review sessions) at your institution when reviewing PE analyses.

The Pharmacoeconomics Canvas

The PE Canvas has three main frames and includes 22 building blocks.

Define the Criteria	**The Question and Objective**	**Perspective**	**Competing alternatives** *options, interventions or comparators*	**Type of Analysis**	**Frame the Methods then Conduct and/or Evaluate the Analysis**	**Conceptual Framework** Design a Conceptual Framework *Structure the decision question and sequence of events for each alternative* Develop an Action Plan *Design the analytical model* *Design the decision model or study method to be used* *The framework and action plan are the basis for the items on the right*	**Model Inputs**	
	Patient Population	**Location**	**Time Horizon**	**Decision Rule or an "Acceptable Threshold"**			Consequences Model inputs: Appropriate **Outcome Measures** Incorporate **Probabilities**	Cost Model inputs: Appropriate **Costs**
Evaluate the Output	**Frame Results** Presentation of the Results (e.g., Title, base case inputs, results, and sensitivity analyses)		**Full Evaluation** What went into the model? What is driving the model? Does it make clinical sense? Where and when can I use this information?				**Resources:** Resources available	**Evidence and Collection of Data**
							Human Resources / Source of data (data source)	Retrieval of Evidence / Data Collection
	Frame Discussion, Recommendation and Conclusion Is it generalizable to your situation? What is the recommendation and how will it inform a decision?						**Adjusting for Time**	**Assumptions**
							Sensitivity Analysis	**Limitations**

Chapter 7: The Pharmacoeconomics Canvas

Pharmacoeconomics Canvas

Define the Criteria

The Question and Objective	Perspective	Competing alternatives *options, interventions or comparators*	Type of Analysis
Patient Population	Location	Time Horizon	Decision Rule or an "Acceptable Threshold"

Frame the Methods then Conduct and/or Evaluate the Analysis

Conceptual Framework

- Design a Conceptual Framework — Structure the decision question and sequence of events for each alternative
- Develop an Action Plan — Design the analytical model
- Design the decision model or study method to be used
- The framework and action plan are the basis for the items on the right

Model Inputs

Consequences Model inputs: Appropriate **Outcome Measures** *Incorporate Probabilities*	Cost Model inputs: Appropriate **Costs**

Resources: Resources available		Evidence and Collection of Data	
Human Resources	Source of data (data source)	Retrieval of Evidence	Data Collection

Adjusting for Time	Assumptions

Sensitivity Analysis	Limitations

Evaluate the Output

Frame Results
Presentation of the Results (e.g., Title, base case inputs, results, and sensitivity analyses)

Full Evaluation
- What went into the model?
- What is driving the model?
- Does it make clinical sense?
- Where and when can I use this information?

Frame Discussion, Recommendation and Conclusion
- Is it generalizable to your situation?
- What is the recommendation and how will it inform a decision?

Frame 1: Define the Criteria

The first frame is to "Define the Criteria" and includes the following building blocks:

Define the Criteria	**The Question and Objective**	**Perspective**	**Competing alternatives** *options, interventions or comparators*	**Type of Analysis**
	Patient Population	**Location**	**Time Horizon**	**Decision Rule or an "Acceptable Threshold"**

At the start of any analysis, you need to define the criteria to the best extent possible so that the readers (i.e., the decision-makers or potential users of the information) can understand the scope of the analysis.[44,77,99,177] Give the reader enough information to understand the context.

You should define the question and objective, perspective, competing alternatives, type of analysis, patient population, location, time horizon, and the decision rule or an "acceptable threshold."

As you build, answer the question: can others replicate this with the information presented? This allows you to assess whether you have provided enough information for the readers.

Block 1 – The Question and Objective

Define a specific, researchable (measurable) question. What question is driving the analysis?

State precisely the two or more competing alternatives you are comparing – for which a decision needs to be made.[1,25,73,77,86,98,99,139,154] Identify the question at hand based on these alternatives or options.

The question and objective must be clear and specific. Be careful not to make the question too narrow – e.g., as a binary decision of yes or no – or keep it way too broad where you will not be able to make a decision. You need it broad enough to describe each alternative. Within the question and objective, include what population the question is relevant to and state the location of the population of interest. The question and objective are the foundation for what you decide will be your outcome measures.[98]

State why this question is important and why it is needed. You will need to be able to articulate what you are hoping to answer with the insights obtained. Make sure the question(s) and objective(s) are relevant to your target audience.

State your hypothesis as part of the introduction. You can either start with the question at hand or start with the population and then build the question around it. For example, you can focus on patients with diabetes and then come to a question, or you can start with a question and then look at the population it affects.

Once you define the other criteria in the frame, you can review your question and edit it accordingly.

No single assessment, checklist, or guidelines will work for every decision question.

Block 2 – Perspective

The question and objective drive the perspective and type of analysis.[41] The perspective taken is often that of decision-makers – those who assess value and ultimately make a decision. Perspective is at the core of any analysis and drives what will be in the model.[1,40,44,53,77,128,138]

Start by answering the following "who" questions:
- Who is your target audience – for whom is this information relevant?
- Who has a connection with the issue at hand?
- Who is likely to face a similar question?
- Who benefits from this information?
- Who are the decision-makers?

Decision-makers vary in preferences, needs, and authority. Creators of these analyses should consider taking multiple perspectives if they want to cast a broader net. Depending on the perspective of the decision-maker of interest and the populations they serve, information may be used differently. Data means different things to different people.

Answer the following questions: What perspective will this study or analysis take? From whose viewpoint are you tackling the question? The choice of the perspective is based on the research question and target audience.

Common Perspectives include:[1,25,41,42,44,53,73,77,98,125,128,139,154]
- Societal
- Health system – e.g., institutional perspective, hospitals, clinics, and providers
- Payer – e.g., insurer
- Healthcare sector
- Patient – with or without family or caregivers'
- Other: e.g., employer, government

The most common perspectives are societal, health system and payer. The gold standard is societal – more on that later.[1,25,41,42,44,53,73,77,98,125,128,139,154]

Remember, perspective matters – it is half the battle.

Choose a perspective based on the audience. The perspective is based on the decision-maker, and the target audience(s) identified. Based on the reader's authority level (power and influence) in decision-making, it may require you to think from multiple perspectives. Consider the various decision-makers' viewpoints on the issue to answer, "What is the other side of the issue?"

You should clearly and explicitly state the perspective of the analysis.[1,25,26,29,40-44,53,73,77,98,125,128,138,139,154]

For example, start the sentence by stating: "The perspective of the study is..."

You can choose any of the numerous perspectives, but state and define the perspective(s) used in the study. A PE study can include more than one perspective, but the results of the different perspective analyses may vary and must be distinctly identified. It is not possible to have one analysis that includes all perspectives.[42]

The societal perspective is the "gold standard" and is often recommended for the reference case.[1,25,41,73,77,98,125,128,139,154] It is considered the most objective since it measures all costs (regardless of who pays them) and benefits (regardless of who receives the benefits) – however, it is difficult to interpret. It is important to note that there is no standard, agreed-upon method for what to include in the societal perspective (both in terms of healthcare and non-healthcare costs).[1,25,41,73,77,98,125,139,154]

Most studies include the health system, payer, or societal perspective.[25,139,154] Although the most appropriate perspective, according to economic theory, is societal, the most common perspective used in PE studies is that of the institution or that of the payer.[25,139,154] The Second Panel on Cost-Effectiveness in Health and Medicine recommends having two perspectives as the reference case (the health sector perspective and the societal perspective), allowing for consistency and comparability across a number of studies.[41,138] It has been recommended to consider including the perspective of those who are paying for the product or services along with the reference case of societal and health sector.[42,77] Criticism around having to include the two perspectives as reference cases still exist, as it may not be relevant to the audience.[77,125] It is up to you to determine which perspective makes the most sense and then pick costs and outcome measures relevant to that perspective.[125] If you are focused on patient-level and shared decision-making among healthcare providers and patients, it is critical to incorporate a patient, family, or caregiver perspective.

Perspective impacts the costs and the outcomes to be included – as well as the decision criteria, time period of the evaluation, decision rules, and the final recommendation(s). When you identify whose perspective you will take, you can then identify relevant costs, outcomes, and model inputs to make appropriate recommendations based on the data. Perspective also drives the interpretation of the results and recommendations.

A PE analysis will be critiqued based on the perspective of the reader. Perspective helps determine what costs are relevant. The choice of perspective primarily drives cost choices.

Consider making the perspective that of your decision-maker and then incorporate costs and outcomes that are relevant to and are of interest to that perspective.[26,53,73,98,125]

Block 3 – Competing Alternatives

The competing alternatives are options, often known as the "comparators." Competing alternatives, options, choices, and comparators are used interchangeably. Start with making a comprehensive list of all the options or competing alternatives available to the patient, given the situation or case. Answer: "what options are available to the patient"? The competing alternatives must be options we see in the real-world. Think of the most commonly used options and what offers clinical benefits.[25,26,29] You can also include a "do-nothing option" or "no intervention" when that is a valid option and makes sense.[77] Carefully assess the options, as there is no need to compare an intervention to an outdated, ineffective intervention.

You should include what is already being done, the standard of care – i.e., "existing practice or therapy" or the "status quo."[25,26,29,44,77] One would generally use the current standard of care as a comparator; since we want to decide between a new product or service compared with what we are currently offering or what is available.[29,44,77] Include the "new option" or the options we have to choose between along with the standard of care. Sometimes you do not have a "new option," but rather, you are assessing the current options available and deciding between them – hence this step is critical as you make the distinction.[1,25,29,73,86]

Examples of options:
- Introducing a new medication to the options list for a particular health condition – thus can compare two medications or a medication to a non-pharmacological treatment option.[73]
- Introducing a new program compared with an existing program for a particular condition.

Choose at least two from these competing alternatives, which you will evaluate. These options need to be "mutually exclusive options" – an "either" "or" situation.[77,99] The options would be replacing each other. You would not be implementing both – it is one or the other – hence they are competing.[29,73] By saying yes to one thing, you would also be saying no to something else – this is **opportunity costs**.[2,42,53,156] For example, when a new technology comes into the market, it replaces the old technology or old practices.

State why you chose those particular options to be evaluated for the decision question. The rationale is important when the lower cost or higher benefit option is not selected.[139,154]

As you evaluate the analyses, you will ask (at the bare minimum): Are the comparators stated?[29]

Clearly define the intervention that is within each option

Describe the intervention – is it a product, service, or program? Be as comprehensive and as specific as possible. Carefully define all the components of the interventions – even items such as location – as they may affect the other elements and outcomes of the interventions. Provide explicit details. The more detail you provide on the options, the better the evaluator of the study can assess whether it is valid or credible and whether they can replicate it.[25] When comparing medications, make sure to be very detailed regarding all aspects of the drug. For example, make sure to state the name of the medication, dosage, dosage schedule, route of administration, duration of treatment, etc.[25,139,154] Distinctly highlight where the innovation is – make a note of it for yourself so that you can speak to it. This is essential to do since you can highlight this in your "why." Alternatively, what you already indicated in your "why" previously can be applied here.

Analyze all competing alternatives in the same way. Consider using a table, such as Table 1, to compare the competing options using similar metrics.[98] This may also assist you in building the case for competing options, support you in describing the competing options, and allow you to focus on what to compare. Examples of Detailed Features of the Product or Service Compare Across Competing Options are shown in Table 2. These tables will allow you to include any items you want to compare between the two or more alternatives.

The choice of competing alternatives primarily drives the outcomes or consequences selections. You should answer the question: "what are your measures of effectiveness?

Table 1: Comparison of Competing Alternatives or Options		
Detailed Features of the Product or Service	**Existing product or service or Standard of care *** **(Name or "0")**	**New product or service (Name or "1")**
List the items you want to compare		

* Option that will be replaced with new product or service

Table 2: Examples of Detailed Features of the Product or Service to Compare Across Competing Options
Characteristics of the product or service: Explain the features of the product or service.
Disease or condition treating
Function of the product or service: What does it do? What are the features?
Unique restriction of the product or service: Outline any unique restriction(s) on how the product or service can be used.
Benefits of the product or service: List the benefits. Consider tailoring it based on perspective, as benefits can mean different things to different people. For each new option, explain: How is the latest product or service different? Is it of value because it is more innovative compared to the current products or services? Does it have added features and attributes compared with the standard of care? Does it produce better outcomes and cost less? Refer to the cost-effectiveness plane to determine which quadrant the new product or service lies compared with standard care.
Potential disadvantages: List any harms or concerns associated with the product or service.
Safety: Briefly explain or summarize the safety of the product or service and then compare it to the competing option. State whether it has a higher or lower safety profile compared with the competing option. May consider using "+/-" or up and down arrows to reflect the meaning.
Efficacy: Briefly explain or summarize the efficacy of the product or service and compare it with the competing option. Clearly define the measure of efficacy here and state whether it has a higher or lower efficacy compared with the competing option for each measure. May even consider going a step further and adding a column for assessing the quality of the evidence.
Cost: Consider adding the actual cost or consider putting a range if you have it. Otherwise, you can also place a "+ or –" compared to the competing option until you find the actual numbers.
Product or service outcomes of interest: Identify what outcomes are applicable. The analysis can determine the types of outcomes, or the consequences can determine the type of analysis. For example, if you know you want to do a cost-benefit or cost-effectiveness analysis (CEA), you choose the appropriate outcome based on each analysis type. Make sure to state the reason for inclusion for those specific outcomes.
Other considerations: Are there any other considerations that should be taken into account? For example, ethical reasons for choosing this intervention (regardless of outcomes).

Block 4 – Type of Analysis

Clearly state the type of analysis. The evaluator should be able to quickly identify the type of analysis to assess whether it was the appropriate or most suitable analysis type. Answer the question: Was the type of PE analysis stated? Was the appropriate type of PE used?[25,29,73,77,177]

The choice of the analysis type is based on the outcome measures in consideration. In other words, the type of analysis depends on the outcome measure assessed.

Comparison Across Economic Analyses

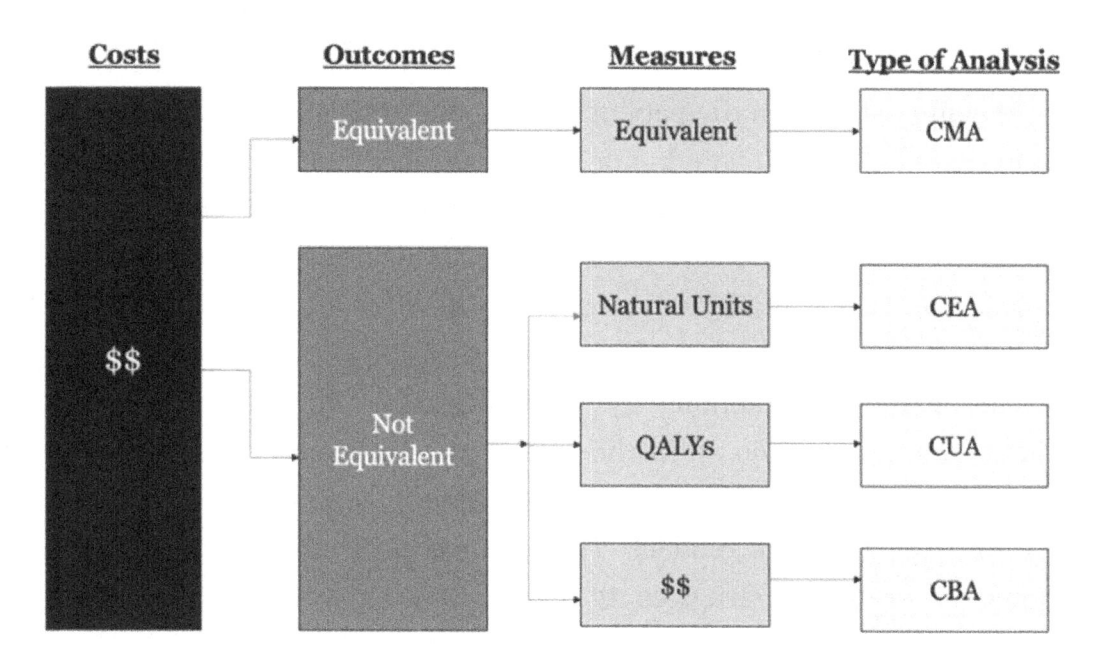

Costs	Outcomes	Measures	Type of Analysis
$$	Equivalent	Equivalent	CMA
$$	Not Equivalent	Natural Units	CEA
$$	Not Equivalent	QALYs	CUA
$$	Not Equivalent	$$	CBA

$$ = dollars or any monetary value; QALYs = quality-adjusted life years; CMA = cost-minimization analysis; CEA = cost-effectiveness analysis; CBA = cost-benefit analysis; CUA = cost-utility analysis [1,2,25,39,43,44,53,73,98,153]

One study or evaluation may perform or contain more than one type of analysis.[29]

Block 5 – Patient Population

The patient population is the population you are interested in ultimately answering the decision question: who is it benefiting? It is the population that is affected by the interventions and within whom you are evaluating these interventions.

Define your target population for the intervention(s)

Define your baseline characteristics **or base-case population**. Base case characteristics can include demographics (e.g., age and gender), the severity of the disease, and risk factors, among many others. Be very specific when defining the patient population and state your rationale for choosing this particular patient population. It may be the specific population you serve, or it may be the patient population seen in the efficacy or effectiveness trials. We often start with the patient population we need to make a decision for and then begin to describe them. If you do not have a specific population in mind, you may consider starting by evaluating the effectiveness trials and literature to see the patient population characteristics in which these interventions were evaluated and then proceed to define yours – however, there are limitations to this approach.

When you define the patient population, try to understand more than just their demographics – think about what could affect the costs and consequences. Carefully note any patient characteristics or factors that may affect the effectiveness or outcome data (e.g., the severity of the disease, age, and gender). Try to understand their needs, various situations, and potential or actual struggles to understand behavior and real-world situations.

Compare patient populations. Compare the patient characteristics you defined in the base case to those found in the literature when looking for studies to extract the effectiveness data.

When conducting PE analyses, you often have to retrieve information from other diverse sources, each with varying patient populations. As you begin to dig deeper into the literature, you need to understand how applicable the current effectiveness data is to your patient population of interest. Establishing a system to compare patient populations early on will help with data collection for any other outcome measures you have identified. You will use this information frequently.

Consider having a table similar to Table 3 when you begin the literature search to compare patient characteristics of those in the various studies. It will assist you in answering the question: is this relevant to your population? It will also help you identify a list of assumptions and limitations in the data you do find – which you will need to be able to speak to later in your discussion.

Table 3: Literature Review Database

Analysis	Literature		
Patient Population of Interest	Name of the study	Patient population characteristics studied	Is this relevant to your population? Justify response
Base Case *Baseline Characteristics of interest* *Ideal patient population* *Similar to inclusion criteria*			Yes — If yes, how? / No — If no, what defers?

Whether you are <u>evaluating or conducting</u>, look at the characteristics of the population, and continuously ask: is this relevant to the population you serve? If so, how? If not, why? Can the differences you noticed be adjusted later in the analyses? Differences in patient characteristics can lead to differences in effectiveness data.[139] Understand if, when, where, and what patient characteristics are driving the effectiveness shown. For example, effectiveness data in patients with less severe disease may have better outcomes than those with high severity levels. Baseline risk affects the potential benefits of the interventions.

The outcome and effectiveness data are established from trials in specific patient populations; thus, it is essential to compare patient population characteristics to ensure you are using the correct data. The data used in the analysis are taken from population averages and do not account for patient heterogeneity.[26,41,138]

If you want to use the information you find in your population, you have to make sure the study population and your population of interest are similar. The studies from which you will extract effectiveness data will often not be your precise population – therefore, you should evaluate whether to use that information or whether you can adjust the differences between the populations later in the analyses.

Block 6 – Location

To further understand the decision-making setting, you must know the location of the population studied. Specify the following items:
- Geographical location – e.g., country, state, and city.
- Type of institution – e.g., private sector, public sector, community-based facilities, health system, clinics, academic, pharmacy benefits management company, or pharmaceutical company.
- Number of institutions – single vs. multiple institutions.
- Where the interventions were provided and evaluated.
- Where and how the resource allocation decisions are being considered or contemplated.

It is critical to recognize where and how decisions are made in that location. Each country and location may vary in the interventions available to them, their definition of value, payment systems, and ultimately how they make decisions.[1,7,26,29,54,88,129-133]

If the countries differ, costs will differ as well.

The location of the population studied, the evaluation process, and the decision-makers will shed light on system-level differences and can determine how generalizable and transferable the information is to your particular setting. It will drive you to understand their decision-making process better – that is, how decisions are made and what choices are implemented in that location.

Block 7 – Time Horizon

Choose the time period for which you will evaluate the costs and consequences of the options. Clearly state the rationale for the choice of the time horizon. The time horizon can vary based on the perspective – e.g., one month, one year, ten years, a lifetime. However, the ideal and most commonly used time horizon is **lifetime**.

The basis for choosing a longer time horizon is the need to capture long-term differences – in benefits and costs – between interventions overall. Many long-term benefits (e.g., reduction in secondary and tertiary events and reduction in hospitalization) and changes in costs (e.g., medications go off patents and become generic, lowering costs of medications) may be seen after a given time period post-intervention (e.g., months to years).[20,44,53,77,86,99,139]

If a lifetime horizon is not chosen, the time horizon should cover a sufficient time period to demonstrate differences in benefits or costs.

Block 8 – Decision Rule or an "Acceptable Threshold"

Once you get the analysis results, what will you do with them? How are you making the decision? How will you use the results to determine your course of action? Will this impact your decision? For example, will you implement a service or introduce a product regardless of the outcome of the analysis? If you know you will apply the intervention – do you care to understand beyond the budget impact? These are critical questions that must be answered before embarking on a PE analysis. What you will do with the information is often a struggle.

You need to be able to clearly articulate why you are conducting this analysis. How do you anticipate the analysis will inform decision-making?

Map out your decision-making process by answering key questions, such as:
- How much are you willing to spend?
- How generous are you?
- How are you making the decision?
- Will this impact your decision?
- How will you use the results to determine your course of action?
- What justification strategy will you use to make your decision?
- "What do you consider good value for your money?"[42] This goes beyond a budget question – it is not just a "can I afford this intervention or program?" question. How much value do you think you are getting?
- Is the extra benefit worth the additional cost?

Decision-makers must be able to articulate what they consider value for money, opportunity costs, and budget constraints.

Decision Rules

The decision that results from this analysis is hard to make. The decision criteria are based on a judgment call – you need to decide if the extra unit of effectiveness is worth the additional cost.[29,73]

Thresholds

One approach to creating a decision rule to assist with coverage and allocation decisions is through the use of a threshold.[42,156] Thresholds can be either implicit or explicit, and different thresholds may be applied for different diseases.[20,26,45,156,188]

Due to the diversity of decision-makers in healthcare, we can see a wide variety of thresholds and decision rules.[20,188] Thresholds are based on the decision-maker and all of their own "criteria" or elements of value. No universal threshold exists that incorporates all decision-maker perspectives.[20,45,189]

There are inconsistencies with the use and choice of different thresholds, if used at all. Everyone chooses different thresholds – as payers, consumers, decision-makers have different willingness-to-pay (WTP) thresholds.[45,156,188,189] Some patients' WTP is above a set threshold.[26,156,189] Payers should consider individual preferences when establishing thresholds.[42]

Keep in mind who is valuing the intervention.
How much a payer is willing to pay often differs from what the patient is willing to pay.

The conventional approach or "central method" is to use a cost-per-quality-adjusted life-year (QALY) metric for a **cost-effectiveness threshold.**[42,45,77,156] The threshold range often seen in the literature of $50,000 to $150,000/QALY is not based on any rigorous analysis.[9,26,45,73,138,156]

More wealthy countries tend to put a higher value on a QALY, but this is not the rule. Thresholds are developed with input from various stakeholders and are based explicitly on country, population characteristics, and preferences.[26,86,188] Thresholds vary among countries, payers, providers, and patients. They may increase over time as the price of technology, products, and services increases and may differ based on disease states.

The value set for the threshold depends on factors such as opportunity costs, budget, and in some cases, preferences of those you serve or represent, and the WTP of consumers.[45] Threshold can be set in relation to opportunity costs or gross domestic product (GDP) in some countries.[39] This is particularly useful to know if or when you begin to compare thresholds across countries.[45,156,190,191]

One must evaluate how an intervention will impact the budget. A low threshold means you are working with a more restrictive budget. Whereas, a higher threshold means you will allow for more options – it is assuming you have a larger budget.[42,156]

Several analyses may not even provide decision criteria or explicitly state whether they are using a threshold in the decision-making process. Determine whether a decision rule or threshold was set and reported.

A limited number of decision-makers use a threshold to inform policy – or at least a few make public statements of their use. Some experts have recommended avoiding the use of a specific threshold to inform policy.[77,122,189] Countries and institutions may even set up policies prohibiting the use of a dollars (cost)-per-QALY threshold in their coverage and allocation decisions.[77,122,189] Decide whether you will use a threshold to inform your decision-making.

If you do set or use a threshold, you should:
- Consider the decision context[77,190]
- Make sure to receive input from other stakeholders
- Avoid using only one specific acceptable threshold, as no single threshold can cover all patient populations, perspectives, and diseases.[9,20,77] It has been recommended to use a range of thresholds rather than one concrete number.[45,77,86]
- Consider it be part of a "multi-criteria decision analysis" – where you also consider other factors and elements.[42] Make the threshold only part of the decision – that is, one input of many in the decision-making process. Rather than using the threshold as a set rule, consider other elements in parallel.
- It should be a starting point and not the final rule, as other factors should be considered. There are several limitations associated with the methodology of incremental cost-effectiveness ratios (ICERs). For example, people question what evidence went into the model, limiting its complete validity as the only decision-making tool.[42,156]

You may consider setting a threshold but be deliberate. Recognize there is ambiguity in decision-making.[41] Even if you decide to set a threshold explicitly, you should examine and determine in what situation you would modify this number. You need to be thoughtful and recognize all the conditions which will change your decision.[60,156]

Clearly define your modifiers. If you set a threshold, in what situation would you modify this number? Define the "modifiers" from your rule – e.g., social justice, disease severity, and equity that may influence your decisions.[42,45,76,156] Involve as many relevant stakeholders as to determine what modifiers require attention.

Frame 2: Frame the Methods then Conduct and/or Evaluate

Let us build off the "Define the Criteria" frame and move to the second frame to conceptualize the analysis further. You will visibly outline and tell the story of the interventions and outcomes using structured methods.

The second frame is "Frame the Methods then Conduct and/or Evaluate the Analysis" and includes the following building blocks:

	Conceptual Framework	Model Inputs	
Frame the Methods then Conduct and/or Evaluate the Analysis	Design a Conceptual Framework	Consequences Model inputs: Appropriate **Outcome Measures** *Incorporate* **Probabilities**	Cost Model inputs: Appropriate **Costs**
	Structure the decision question and sequence of events for each alternative Develop an Action Plan	**Resources:** Resources available || **Evidence and Collection of Data**	
		Human Resources	Source of data (data source)	Retrieval of Evidence	Data Collection
	Design the analytical model	**Adjusting for Time**	**Assumptions**
	Design the decision model or study method to be used *The framework and action plan are the basis for the items on the right*	**Sensitivity Analysis**	**Limitations**

156

Block 9 – Design a Conceptual Framework

Design and build a conceptual framework around the competing alternatives for the model. Here you will define or map out the pathways for the interventions you have identified to help you determine what needs to be captured or collected. This is where you look at the process as a system of parts.

The conceptual framework block is on the left with a dotted line to all the items it includes on the right. In other words, you should incorporate the blocks on the right in your conceptual framework. The framework and action plan in the block are the groundwork for the blocks on the right.

The framework should include a detailed sequence of events for each alternative.[1,2,25,29,43,44,53,73,77,98,99]

Structure the decision question and series of events for each alternative – that is, the events that will occur as a result of each intervention. Start by answering: What do you know at this moment to be true about the interventions and the associated outcomes?

To create the pathways and determine the appropriate outcomes, you should be aware of the natural course of the disease or the patients' condition. Written and visual methods (e.g., in the form of figures) can assist with summarizing the health condition and associated health states for this activity.[77]

Not only should you ask what are the outcomes, but what are causing the consequences? You want your model to reflect what happens as a result of the interventions or alternatives. Include the outcomes achieved and the relationship between all the factors causing the outcomes. As your building the framework, make a note of what may influence your model.

Similar to the first frame, as you map out processes, consider documenting where the unique innovation is of the new intervention (if it exists) so you are aware and able to speak about it.

Concept 1: Develop an Action Plan

The action plan is where you chart your roadmap for the analysis. It requires strategic foresight, organization, and creating your own checklists – using resources like the PE Canvas. Be proactive and develop a detailed action plan that will help you define all components of your analysis.

Developing an action plan requires defining the steps, resources, and people needed for the actual analysis. The plan is where you tell the audience what you included in the assessment. This includes why you added what you did and where it is from (or its source). Overall, it contains what goes into the analysis and the process you took or will take to conduct it.

The action plan will summarize how you plan to implement the methods you indicate.

Create an action plan for **each block in the frame.** Outline the **design features** of the analysis to compare it to others when you retrieve the information and evaluate other analyses. Consider creating a process flowchart – your internal plan to live by – one that can be unique to yourself or your institution. You can also use the suggestions in **The Process section** from Chapter 6.

The actual approach you decide to take may be unique to your institution, but it can also be influenced by the question at hand, time, the perspective of the analysis, and the number of resources required (e.g., data sources, financial resources).[29]

You will be answering the following questions to outline the components of the analysis:
- What items are or will be included in the model or analysis?[77,99] Distinctly describe how you went about estimating the parameters (e.g., transition probabilities).[139]
- Where will you obtain your data? How credible is the data?
- What are the variables – both dependent and independent? Identify relevant variables in terms of costs and outcomes in the analysis.
- How do you measure the variables? And why did you use that approach?[77,99]
- Clearly articulate what you have decided to include and what you chose to exclude.

Be sure to determine and clearly describe the methods you are using.[86]

Define a plan for dealing with any "problem" data or data that is missing or may not directly extrapolate to your patient population. How will you account for the heterogeneity of the data (population-level data that are an aggregate of average responses vs. individual variations)?[20,26,53,139,177] How will you respond to uncertainty in the data?

After you map it all out, determine your collective focus – where will you invest the most time and effort? Identify what information is the hardest and easiest to obtain. Allocate the appropriate time for each of these. Spend most of your time and resources on the hardest items or items that take the longest to obtain.

Apply metrics, milestones, and specific delivery dates to each item to both track progress and hold yourself accountable. Set measurable goals and track progress metrics that matter. Create methods to keep track of everything and develop a process to double-check your work. Decide what sort of documentation you want to keep. Documentation forms for data collection may be helpful and can be built based on the needs. Consider creating templates and incorporating them into the workflow.

Determine a method(s) for obtaining the information you need to evaluate the interventions. Decide if you want to conduct studies to collect the data you need for your model or if you want to extract the data that is available in the literature. In other words, will you perform these study designs and methods to generate the input variables, or will you retrieve them from the literature? Some may consider doing both – collecting and retrieving. Each option has its strengths and limitations, and you can speak to each when you evaluate your results and in the discussion of the analysis. The choice of the method can also depend on or be influenced by how much time, money, and resources are available to you.[29] The important thing is to choose a method – be clear as to which method(s) you are selecting – and then plan accordingly.[139,154]

There are several approaches, tools, and designs used in PE to obtain the data needed to inform a decision.[1] There are practice standards but no standard methods or one set of rules.[29]

Examples of various **study designs** used in outcomes research include randomized controlled trials, cohort studies, case-control studies, case reports, case series, systematic reviews, meta-analysis, retrospective claims analysis, mixed design (e.g., data collection as well as data generated from clinical trials) and **decision analysis.**[1,20,26,28,29,40-45,53,73,77,86,99,109,139,154,177,192]

You can either "directly" conduct the studies using randomized control trials (a controlled environment), naturalistic trials, resemble clinical practice, observational data (trials or claims data) or conduct decision analysis when resource limitation factors are present – i.e., limited time and money to directly collect the data.[43,44,73,109] Explore what information is out there. Use a systematic approach to find the information and define a strategy of what data and data sources you will use.

Strive for transparency

Transparency is principal, as the results and use of the analysis results are judged based on the methods used. Be transparent in how, what, where, why you choose the values and items you included.[1,20,26,28,29,40-45,53,73,77,86,99,109,139,154,177,192] Those reading the analysis must have sufficient information to reproduce it. You will also be evaluated on the ease of reproducing the analysis.

Transparency of items such as the audience, perspective, design and methods, decision criteria, assumptions, and data sources is critical.[40,42,45] You may be required to provide all the details of the analysis to reviewers. Hence, make transparency essential among your team to facilitate external transparency. Discussions remain as to how much is needed to share for the sake of publications due to the intellectual property of that model.[28]

Concept 2: Decision Analysis

Decision analyses are used when there is uncertainty regarding the decision between competing alternatives.[1,2,25,44,53,73] All the needed data is often not available all in one study; therefore, simulations and retrieval of data from the literature may become warranted.

With decision analyses, you create a hypothetical situation or model to answer the question at hand.[1,2] Since it is a hypothetical situation, you are not performing the study to get the data – but instead, you are collecting the data from the available literature.[1] This method is often used when you cannot collect all the data you need, or the data does not exist in one trial to make a decision.[73] You combine data from multiple sources into a structure model that resembles the sequence of events that occur as a result of each competing alternative. What is particularly appealing about this approach is that it helps systematically tell a story of the events resulting from choosing a specific intervention. You must identify the competing alternatives to which a decision needs to be made, structure the sequence of events for each option, and incorporate probabilities.[1,2,25,29,44,98] It allows you to assign both costs and probabilities to each event. List all possible outcomes (both positive and negative) and decide what to include based on the perspective.

A chief advantage of decision analysis is that it can evaluate multiple factors and allows for the integration of elements that assess the effectiveness of an intervention and not just efficacy and safety.[1,2] The use of decision analysis depends on the type of analysis – as it is commonly used for CEA or CUA.[1,2,25,29,44,98]

Design the analytical model

There are several simulations and decision modeling methods available.[2,53,77,139,154,193,194] Choose between them and provide the rationale for why it was chosen. Make sure to explain why it is appropriate for this analysis.[73,139,154]

Two frequently used **decision models** in the literature include decision-analytic models (decision tree) and Markov models.[2,44,53,73,77,138,139,154,193,194] The disease for which the interventions are used often determines which decision models to choose.[1] More than one model can be used together. Depending on the health condition assessed, you may consider having two models in the analysis.[1,73,77,99]

A simple summary of steps for the decision models includes:[1,2,25,29,43,44,53,73,77,87,98,99]

1. Draw the decision model structure (e.g., decision tree or Markov model), which will portray your sequence of events. Make a list of all possible outcomes – both positive and negative – and decide what to include based on the perspective.
2. Add probabilities to each event or outcome, or consequence. The probability is the "chance" or "likelihood" of that event occurring. Find and add estimated probabilities to the events to obtain the expected value.
3. Add or specify costs to each event or outcome, or consequence.
4. Perform the calculations for each decision. Clearly summarize any calculations made – no matter how simple they may seem.
5. Analyze the results to make a recommendation(s) that can help inform a decision.
6. Test for uncertainty and robustness of the model by performing sensitivity analyses.
7. Ensure you state what modeling or method you used and if you used any software to create the model.

Decision Tree

A decision tree is the most common, simple way to frame the pathways and visually describe the model structure.[1,2,25,44,53,73] Decision trees provide a graphic representation of the competing alternatives, the outcomes associated with each option from start to finish and incorporates the probabilities of those outcomes occurring to draw the path a patient travels.[1,2,25,53,139,154]

Simply put, a decision tree starts with the decision or choice node, incorporates the sequence of events at various chance or probability nodes (driven by probability), and ends with a terminal node.[1,2,25,44,53,73]

Simple Decision Tree

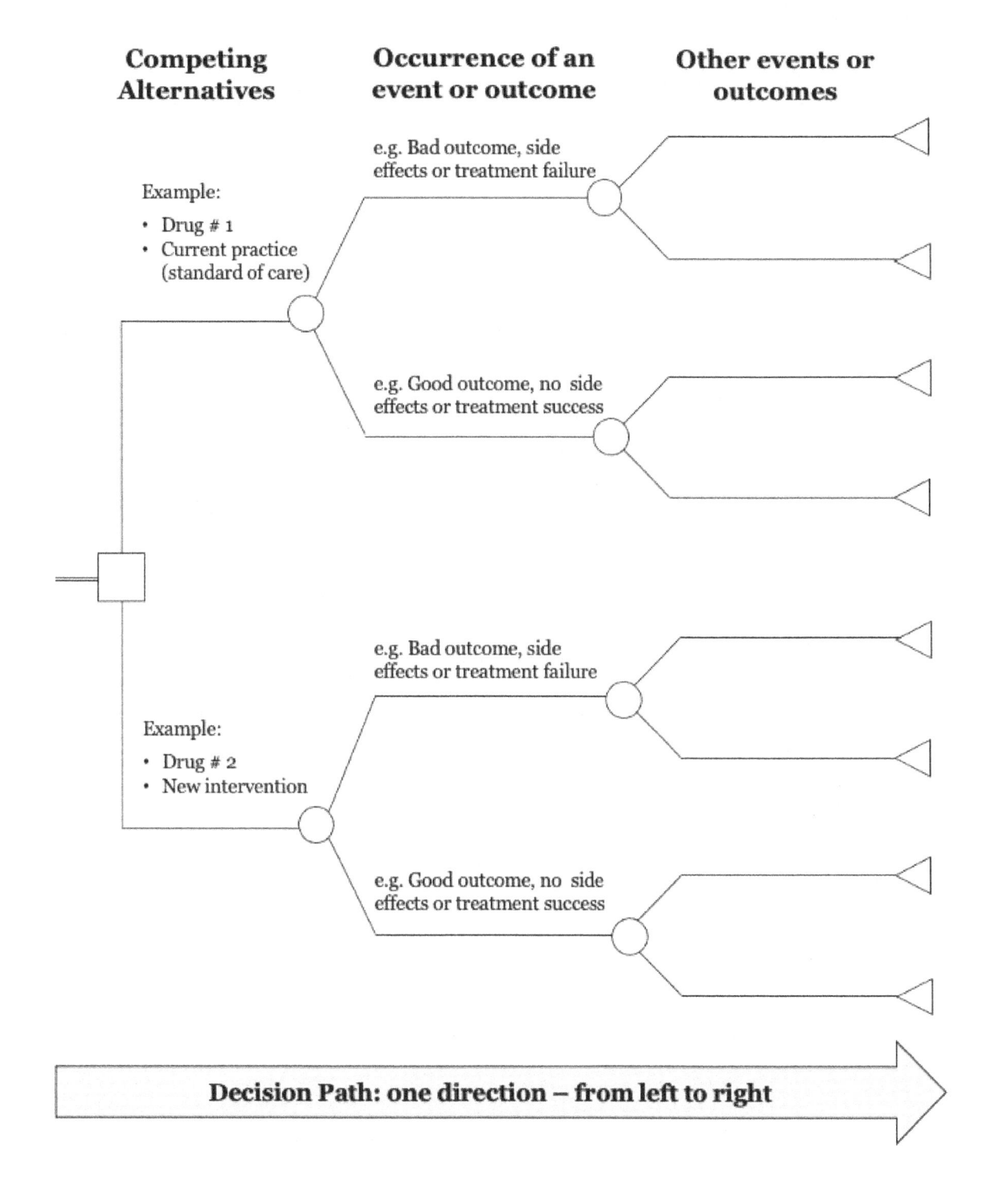

Competing Alternatives

Example:
- Drug # 1
- Current practice (standard of care)

Example:
- Drug # 2
- New intervention

Occurrence of an event or outcome

e.g. Bad outcome, side effects or treatment failure

e.g. Good outcome, no side effects or treatment success

e.g. Bad outcome, side effects or treatment failure

e.g. Good outcome, no side effects or treatment success

Other events or outcomes

Decision Path: one direction – from left to right

Square - decision node or "choice node"[1,2,25,44,53,73] The point in a decision tree at which a decision must be made between the competing alternatives is the decision node or choice node. The decision-maker has control here. The decision-maker has to decide which alternative or option to choose. For example, they could be deciding between at least two medications, two treatments, two services, or interventions. A decision has to be made between the alternatives to move forward. The choice decides the sequence of events to follow. It starts with the graphical representation of the question at hand. For example, if the decision is to treat, the process follows the tree branch for drug therapy.[73] A branch connects the decision node to a chance or probability node.

Branches start from a node and represent the pathway – or the "event" or "consequence" that occurs or the event of interest – to the next node, where another branch leads to an event.[1,2,44,98] For each branch, assign a probability, outcome measure or effects (e.g., utility) and cost to each event. When you draw the tree and add the probabilities to the branches, you assume that the products do not differ in any aspect other than shown in the tree – unless you state this in the limitation section and account for it in your sensitivity analysis.

Circle – chance or probability node:[1,2,25,44,53,73] The events or outcomes that occur after a chance node depends on probabilities.

Triangle – terminal node: A terminal node is placed after the "final" outcome. It is called the "final" outcome since the patients cannot progress past a terminal node.[2,25,44,53,73]

Limitations

You have to keep the decision tree simple. You cannot add a branch for every single possible event. The pathway only travels from left to right in one direction and does not allow for movement back and forth.[1,2] This is especially important when it comes to complex disease states.[1] Decision trees are not ideal to use for chronic disease states that may have multiple events and relapses or conditions that do not follow a single direction.[2,73]

Markov Models

Markov models are often used to reflect the changes in health states associated with chronic disease – where the natural progression of the disease involves a mix of healthier and potentially worsen health.[1,2,29,44,53,73] Patients can either improve, worsen, or stay the same throughout the progression of the disease.

For Markov models, you need to determine health states, transition probabilities, and model cycles.

Health States

A basic Markov model has three health states: well, dead or ill.[1,2,53,73] One can transition back and forth between the health states, except when they transition to "dead."[1,73] "Death" is considered an "absorbing state," and the person does not transition to another health state. Choose the health states that best reflect the disease and outcomes you are evaluating.[29] Add various health states – such as secondary health events like secondary stroke, heart attack, heart failure – depending on the health condition or disease. Calculate costs associated with each health state. Determine the outcomes related to each health state – e.g., utility in that health state.

Transition Probabilities

Classify how and to what health state the patient can transition to and then identify the transition probabilities between each health state.[1,2,29,53,73]

Model Cycle

Each model is run in cycles. Determine how long you would like that cycle to be, e.g., one year, five years, etc., and make sure to account for time differences when appropriate.[1,2,29,53,73]

Blocks 10 and 11 – Model Inputs

	Model Inputs *Identify and outline model inputs*	
Frame the Methods then Conduct and/or Evaluate the Analysis	Consequences Model inputs: Appropriate **Outcome Measures** *Incorporate* ***Probabilities***	Cost Model inputs: Appropriate **Costs**

Identify, Outline and Measure Model Inputs

Model inputs are estimates of all the resources used and the outcome measures associated with each intervention.[25,29,73] Model inputs should "capture the effects" – in terms of costs and outcomes – of interventions in the real-world.[42,43]

Make a list of all possible outcomes (both positive and negative) and decide what to include, tailored to the perspective. Specify all the relevant costs and outcome measures of interest. This consists of all associated costs of each alternative and the outcome valued in whatever units of interest (e.g., utility for QALYs). Choose and value the relevant cost and outcome inputs.[25,26,29,43,73,77,99] The more detail you have outlined regarding what went into the model, the easier it is to determine if the relevant costs and consequences were included.[25,177]

Carefully review all model inputs to determine if all relevant and appropriate costs, resources, and outcomes were used.[1]

Costs and outcomes data come from several sources; therefore, each model input's data sources should be outlined in the summary of the analysis.[80] The chances of finding data for every possible cost and consequence are rare; therefore, prioritize the significant ones.[25,77,99]

Justify the use of specific costs and outcomes whenever possible.[25,29] If some costs and outcomes are relevant to the interventions, but you did not include them, you must explain the reason(s) for exclusion.[25] Even a simple statement is beneficial, indicating that the data was not available or was difficult to obtain.[29] The reader may disregard your finding because they may feel that you do not understand or see the full picture.

The estimates we put into our model are part of the **base-case** or the **baseline estimates**. We vary the numbers or estimates of the base-case using sensitivity analysis to determine the "robustness" of the model – to answer, "how sensitive is the model to changes in the values?" If you adjust any of the numbers in the data collection phase, make sure to describe what you did and why.

Block 10 – Consequences Model Inputs: Appropriate Outcome Measures

The outcome measures are the estimates that you will collect data on to demonstrate the effectiveness of an intervention.[1] The outcome measures are meant to resemble or portray the benefits and consequences of an intervention.[139] The choice of outcome measures is selected based on the study question and perspective or intended audience of the analysis.[42,125] The type of analysis is dependent on the outcome measure of interest, but also, the outcome measure you use depends on the kind of analysis you picked. You may have chosen either one first – that is, your outcome determined your analysis type, or your analysis type specified your outcome measures. See Block 4 to walk through the types of analysis.

List all relevant outcome measures associated with each intervention – including both positive and negative consequences.[1,29,44,53,73,77,99] You would have briefly done this previously in the "Define the Criteria" frame, so refer back to it.

Outcomes are multifaceted, there are several to choose from, and some are simpler than others to measure and value.[1,25,29,44]

Examples of outcome measures of interventions to include are clinical and humanistic.
- **Clinical outcomes** are endpoints such as increased life-years saved, reduction in mortality, reduction in morbidity, reduction in cases or cases averted, cure rates, reduction of time to occurrence of secondary conditions such as heart attack, physiologic measures (e.g., hemoglobin A1C), and symptom-free days.[1,25,29,44,73,125]
- **Humanistic outcomes** are endpoints such as a change in the quality of life measures, patient satisfaction, emotional and functional health status, and reduction in symptoms.[1,25,29,44,73]

Negative consequences can include increased morbidity due to drug interactions, adverse events, and increased use of other healthcare resources – e.g., hospital admissions.[1,25,29,44,73,77,99]

Be critical of how you evaluate the outcomes literature. Determine if the outcome measures are final clinical endpoints (e.g., clinical resolution or cure) or surrogate endpoints (e.g., reduced or normalized blood pressure). Since some outcomes take a considerable amount of time to develop and measure, consider using intermediate or surrogate outcomes (e.g., changes in cholesterol levels) when primary or final outcomes (e.g., cure of disease or prevention of heart attack) are challenging to obtain due to the time of follow-up or resources (costs) required to obtain.[9,29,73] Evaluate the **time period** for which the outcomes analyses were conducted and whether that time was sufficient to determine the outcome.[29]

Once you have made a list, determine which outcomes are relevant based on the perspective of the analysis and type of analysis.[73,77,99] Based on what you know about the intended audience, the outcome measures should be relevant to them – that is, clinicians may be more familiar with clinical outcomes such as cases averted compared with QALYs. They must also make clinical sense.[29,125] Be sure to note and explain whether any outcomes were excluded from the analysis.[73,77,99]

Probabilities

You need to find and incorporate the probability or frequency of each outcome.[25] Add probabilities to the events to obtain the expected value. Probabilities should reflect the frequency of occurrence of an event-specific to individuals or populations of interest and are based on evidence.[1,2,53,73,77,99,139,154]

Incorporating Preferences

"Utility" weights are often used to incorporate preferences. Utility is commonly measured on a scale from 0 (representing "dead") to 1 (representing "perfect" health).[29,44,53,73]

Sources that are frequently recommended for preference measures include:
- Community preferences[77,99]
- Generic preference-based measures – e.g., EuroQol 5D (EQ-5D), Short Form 6D (SF-6D), and Quality of Well-Being (QWB).[2,29,43,44,53,73,77,99,153]

Although QALYs is the most accepted measure, its use is not mandatory since it does not capture all consequences of interventions that may be relevant to the intended audience.[42,77]

Block 11 – Cost Model Inputs: Appropriate Costs

Costs are "all the resources used and valued in monetary terms."[77,99]

The general guidance for identifying and outlining the cost inputs include:

1. Make a full **list of all possible costs**. Identify all the resources expended by the interventions over the time period or time horizon you selected.[1,73,77,99,101] For example, the costs associated with outpatient services, inpatient services, and medications over the course of treatment.[1] You care about both present and future costs.

When you start listing the costs, make sure to note the following during the course:
   - Timeframe or date of the estimated cost.[29,139]
   - Currency used in the estimate from the source, and then the currency exchange to the location of where you will implement the intervention or your location.[77,99,139]
   - Any adjustments to the costs and what was done. For example, if you adjusted the cost estimate from the reported year to the current year or converted currency.[139] The year should be consistent across the board for all cost data used.
   - The source of the information.[29]

2. Mark which costs are most relevant to the **perspective**. Ask yourself the question for each cost listed: Does your audience care about this cost? What costs do they endure, and what costs are important to them?[1,25,73] Which costs to consider for inclusion depends on the perspective.[44] The costs need to closely and accurately represent the decision-maker's costs or whose perspective you are targeting.[20,29] Determine whether the target audience bears all the costs now or whether it cost them later. There are upfront costs and the cost savings or "cost offsets" associated with interventions – both at the moment of implementation and into the future.[42] All of these must be considered. "Cost offsets" are reductions in costs later down the road due to long-term improvements (e.g., reduced hospitalizations).[20]

3. **Count** how much is used or the count of occurrence of the event. This is how many times a resource is used, such as the number of office visits.[1,73] If you are conducting an analysis from the societal perspective, make sure not to double count items.

4. **Quantify** this into a monetary value, often done based on the opportunity cost or "next best use."[1,73]

Depending on where you get the cost information from, you may see a variety of costs.[101,139,154,195-197] In situations where the cost is debated (this is most often the case when determining societal costs) consider clearly defining how the cost was calculated. Costs are not the same as charges, as what is charged is not what it ends up costing the user.[73,98] If this is an <u>internal analysis</u>, consider using your cost data whenever possible and available.

<u>Costs based on perspective</u>

Perspective drives what costs to include in the analysis.[1,25,29,73,77,99,139,154] Societal-level perspective is all-inclusive; it incorporates costs to everyone (e.g., healthcare systems patients, insurance companies, families, and society as a whole), as well as costs outside of healthcare (e.g., productivity, child-care, and travel expenses).[1,25,42,73,77,98,99]

The healthcare sector perspective assesses costs associated with the healthcare sector only – e.g., cost of healthcare services and does not include other societal costs such as productivity.[77,98]

This is critical and worth repeating:
make sure the inputs apply to the perspective you have identified.

<u>Types of Costs</u>

Various recommendation task forces provide additional information on the types of costs you can include and the resources used for certain scenarios specifically.[1,25,29,42,44,53,73,77,98,99,101,138] For example, cost data can be obtained from Centers for Medicare and Medicaid Services (CMS) reimbursement rates, various coding systems for physician visits, and average wholesale prices, and use of cost/charge ratios to adjust charge data.[1,25,29,42,44,53,73,77,98,99,101] The four main types of costs include direct medical costs, direct non-medical costs, indirect costs, and intangible costs. Examples for each are shown in Table 4.

Table 4: Types of Costs

Direct medical costs	**Direct non-medical costs**
All the healthcare resources directly consumed by the delivery of the interventions evaluated, including addressing any side effects. Begin with these since they are more prominent and are associated with the resources frequently used in providing healthcare. These include costs associated with: • Medications • Procedures – e.g., x-rays, ultrasounds • Healthcare personnel time • Physicians' visits and services • Medical care • Hospitalizations, room charges, emergency visits • Outpatient visits – e.g., visit to primary care providers and specialists • Laboratory and diagnostics services • Devices and medical equipment – e.g., medical devices such as wheelchairs, hearing aids, pacemakers • Services – e.g., home care, nursing care • Adverse drug reactions	The resources directly consumed by providing the interventions evaluated, however, are considered non-healthcare resources. These include costs associated with: • Transportation – e.g., public or private transportation to and from the healthcare facilities, physician office or hospital, ambulances • All the expenses related to travel, including food and lodging • Daycare or babysitting for children – both formal and informal • Special diets, equipment, or particular changes in their homes to accommodate health conditions Patients and their families often have to endure these costs, as insurance companies or payers usually do not cover such costs.
Indirect costs	**Intangible costs**
These are indirect costs endured by patients, families, caregivers, employers, governments, and societies as a whole. The variability in the indirect costs and how to calculate each cost is the reason no gold standard method exists for calculating these costs. These include costs associated with: • Absenteeism – e.g., employee absences from work due to health condition • Reduced productivity at work or home • Lost productivity due to premature death • Social services – e.g., caregiver and family time	These costs are the most difficult to measure as they represent unquantifiable pain and suffering costs due to the disease or its treatment. Quality of Life (QOL) instruments are often used to reflect patients' health status, utility, and preferences. **Tangible** costs are the direct and indirect costs discussed in the other boxes.

Sources: 1,25,29,42,43,44,53,73,77,98,99,101,138

Block 12 and 13: Resources

	Resources: Resources available	
Frame the Methods then Conduct and/or Evaluate the Analysis	Human Resources	Source of data (data source)

The next two blocks go over where you will get the data you need and who will obtain, create, or review it. You have already determined which key outcomes to measure; now map out the resources to find them. These analyses are resource-intensive and take up a considerable amount of time to conduct.

There are multiple "channels" for information; however, you may not have access to all these outlets.

You will need to answer two questions:
- What crucial resources do you need? Define what resources are required early to assist with the task at hand.
- What resources do you have available to you? Identifying what resources are available to you is instrumental in obtaining the needed information.

Identify both internal and external resources available to you. Do you have your own data to use? If you do not have time and money to collect your own data, you need to use existing evidence. Determine what you can do with what resources you have available to you. Think about time and money. Once you've identified your resources, you can assess whether additional funding is needed.

The limitations of the data sources affect the validity of the results of the analysis.

Block 12 – Human Resources

Be able to describe your team and what they can bring to the table. More information on identifying requirements, team members' skill sets, and the need to delegate appropriately can be found in Chapter 6, Building the Team.

Block 13 – Sources of Data (Data Sources)

You have identified what information to obtain (what input variables are needed), and now, you need to determine how and where to find the appropriate data or evidence. Use the data sources that are most suitable for the measures you have defined.

You will need to answer the following questions:
- Where do I find the data I need?
- For what is the data often used? Answering this can help determine what data source makes the most sense and whether it is appropriate for your needs.
- Is the data or data source credible? You must understand the source of the data and determine if the data is reliable and makes sense – both in practice and methodologically.[139,154]

Review of Literature to Find Model Inputs

There are many data sources available; therefore, it is instrumental that you take some time to determine both what is available to you and decide what you plan to use. The evidence retrieval process is intertwined here.

Data Sources

Sources of costs and outcomes are derived from literature, national and commercial datasets, and expert opinion. Each source of data comes with its limitations, and you must consider this when interpreting the results and applying them to the model. The probabilities used in the model are often taken from the published primary literature and expert opinion.[1,73,139,154]

Information sources include primary (e.g., randomized controlled trials), secondary (e.g., PubMed), and tertiary (e.g., textbook) resources.[25]

Potential data sources include:[1,2,7,20,26,29,43,53,73,95,96,109,115,199,203]
- Published literature
- Clinical trials – e.g., randomized control trials
- Post-marketing trials
- Observational trials and databases
- Retrospective databases
- Medical and prescription claims databases

- Patient registries
- Electronic medical records
- More subjective sources, such as expert opinion
- Unpublished data. If unpublished data is used, the methods to obtain that data should be discussed.
- There may be real-world data (you have or may have collected) that is beyond what is already published.
- Institutional data or your internal data collection.

No single resource will contain everything that is needed for a model.

Blocks 14 and 15 – Evidence and Collection of Data

Block 13 gave you an expansive birds' eye view of potential sources of data; however, now you need to find the data. How do you find the evidence to input into your model? The best, most updated evidence available should inform what you put into the model.[26,43,77,99,112] While the quality of that evidence can significantly vary, it should be informed by evidence, nonetheless.

Block 14 – Retrieval of Evidence

The retrieval of evidence is the multifaceted process by which you obtain the estimates for your model input variables.

Professionals will need to learn how to leverage various types of data to articulate the outcomes and value of a product and intervention. Therefore, you must build the skills to conduct literature and systematic reviews. There are several resources available that guide individuals on how to conduct a systematic review and meta-analysis.[1,2,26,77,99,112,200-207]

Generally speaking, you have to:
1. Identify what you need.
2. Find and assess what is out there.
3. Evaluate the quality of the data.
4. Decide whether you are going to use it in your analysis.[112]

Once you have identified your optimal measures to be used in the model, you should then find the estimates. When conducting or evaluating an analysis, the goal should always be to include the best available evidence.[20]

Clearly articulate your strategy for finding the evidence. Describe the exact process you took to retrieve the studies, how you evaluated those studies, and what information you used.[2,26,139] It would help you outline how you went about appraising, reviewing the literature, and retrieving pertinent data in a transparent and organized manner.[20] Describe what criteria you used in your search and how you determined the eligibility of the studies you decided to review. Whatever method you use to extract the data for the input estimates, make sure you clearly state what you did and the limitations of such a strategy.

State the source of information. Designate your sources of information – e.g., is it from published literature or your own analysis? Many PE studies use data from randomized controlled trials (RCT) and expert opinions into their models.[29] When retrieving and evaluating the studies, differentiate what studies are from RCTs vs. real-world studies – recognizing that both are valuable.

Evaluate the evidence. Now you need to appraise and interpret the data you have found critically.[26,77,112] Many checklists and resources exist summarizing how to go about evaluating literature.[2,7,26,43,44,53,70,71,112,113,139,154,168,203,206-212]

Frameworks and guidelines are available to critique the quality of the evidence.[43,77] The specific criteria for evaluation can vary based on the study design and organization. When you evaluate the evidence, you should state what method you used – e.g., did you use a specific tool? If so, state the tool and definitions of each quality level or category used by that tool.[2,43,77]

When evaluating the data, answer the following questions:
- Is the patient population appropriate?
- Are the interventions appropriate?
- Does it reflect what should be done or seen in practice? Clearly articulate the details of the criteria these studies used. Similar to the first frame and blocks in the canvas, what are the criteria they used?
- Was the study design appropriate? Summarize the study design used to generate the data you retrieved. Consider a table or template to track such information.
- Are the statistical methods appropriate?
- Do they meet any reporting guidelines? Make sure details of outcome measures are stated according to any reported guidance of outcomes.[139,154,213] For example, in a CEA, the method to determine the outcome (often QALYs) must be clearly stated.

The PE Canvas blocks guide you in determining what elements you may need for your model and the items to evaluate other studies.

Summarize the evidence. Define what evidence is available and what is not. Outline the gaps in the literature you noticed and how you accounted for them.

What happens when you can't find the evidence?
When no objective evidence exists, consider using expert opinions. Keep in mind that expert opinions are subjective and may be biased.

Various studies may have **conflicting data** for the same condition or situation – therefore, you should decide what to do when studies conflict.[20]

When synthesizing the evidence, answering the following questions:
- Are the model input estimates based on one study? If so, is this sufficient? Are there any other studies out there? Add justification for the use of only one study.[139,154] If there are multiple studies and you need to combine, consider meta-analysis techniques, when appropriate.[20]
- How do you anticipate extrapolating the results found to your base case scenario?[139,154]

Questions that you should consider when collecting data are:
- How much information are you willing to have to make a decision?
- Would you only confirm the decisions you make with evidence?
- How much data is too much or too little?
- When should you stop collecting the information?
- What do we not know?
- How much uncertainty in the information are you willing to accept?
- Is there such a thing as the "perfect" data?
- Is the extra data worth the added time? What if that data is not available? You may waste time and money trying to find it. You have to make a judgment call on this one.

The responses to these questions may vary based on the "doer" and "user." Descriptions of the "doer" and "user" can be found in Chapter 5.

Block 15 – Data Collection

The data collection process can vary depending on whether you collect the data as part of a study versus collecting data points from the literature. Collecting your own data (in the form of a study) allows you the advantage of obtaining actual numbers within your population of interest – rather than the estimates of other populations in the literature.[25] You will likely find yourself obtaining information from a full array of sources to acquire the best quality and most tailored to your population of interest.

Comparison Across the Studies Retrieved

Summarize the population evaluated in these studies to determine whether this information applies to your target population. The more you can compare the studies' population to your own, the better you are able to assess the relevance of the data into your model.

Consider using a standardized form (or data collection sheets) to extract study details and input estimates from those studies. See Table 5 and Table 6 for an example of a data collection forms you can use across studies and model inputs. These days such "forms" are often created and stored electronically. It may help you extract and track the input estimates from each study you will later include in your model.

Note any adjustments or modifications to the data as you put it into your model. Did you take the input estimates precisely as they were from the source, or did you manipulate them or adjust them in any way to account for differences? Are you taking data from a single study source, multiple sources combined (e.g., meta-analysis), or are you combining the data yourself? If you modified them in any way, you must describe your methods and the rationale for the adjustment and techniques you used.

Base-case estimates are the initial inputs you place into the model before your test for uncertainty. The base case criteria can be used to formulate the study population of interest and study design or features of interest. If your base case is for a lifetime horizon – the studies in which you are extracting data from (e.g., in the case of RCTs) usually do not use such a long time horizon. Therefore, pay close attention to how you are extrapolating the data here and be sure to provide the rationale for your approach.[139,154]

Table 5: Data Collection for Each Study for Comparison Across Studies

Study	Details referencing the study – e.g., title, authors, journal, year.
Year	Add the year of the study to evaluate how updated, and relevant the information is to you and/or your analysis.
Study Design	Indicate whether it is a single-study, multi-study, review article, or meta-analysis (or others when applicable). Evaluate whether the study design is appropriate.
Statistical Methods	Evaluate whether appropriate statistical methods were used.
Limitations (e.g., bias)	Determine what bias exists – e.g., publication bias, selection bias. How was bias handled? State whether you can correct or account for these biases in the model.
Quality	Specify the quality of the study and the method to determine said quality.

Table 6: Data Collection for Each Model Input Estimates

Measures to collect	Define a measure(s). Include the model input estimates.
Estimates from the Evidence	Write down the input estimates exactly how they appear in the literature. Make sure to note if the estimates came from more than one study – i.e., from a meta-analysis.
Adjusted Estimates	Applicable to include when you have adjusted the estimate. Specify the method and reasoning for adjusting the estimate.[77,99]
Data Sources	State the data source – e.g., published literature. Be specific.
Justification for Use	Justify the use of this information or data source.[1,77,99]
Limitations of the data that exist (e.g., in data, model, criteria, methods, etc.)	Limitations will shed light on where sensitivity analyses need to be performed. Keep note of these as you retrieve the evidence to understand the limitations of the evidence and determine whether these shortcomings could potentially influence your model. Make sure to disclose what you did or plan to do to address the limitations during data collection.

Block 16: Adjusting for Time

Since costs and outcomes associated with interventions may appear at different points in time (past, present, and future), you cannot add all the costs and outcomes without accounting for these differences.[1] The money you have today is worth more than the money you have one year (and subsequent years) from today.[1] You have to account for differences in costs and benefits in different time periods and overtime.[29,44,73]

Discounting

Future costs and outcomes must be discounted to their present value to compare the competing alternatives at this point accurately.[1,77,98,99]

How to tell whether you need to discount?
- If you evaluate the costs and outcomes of competing alternatives for less than or equal to (≤) one year and assume the expenses occur at the beginning of the first year, there is no need to discount.[25,139,154]
- When cost and outcomes data of competing alternatives are evaluated for more than (>) one year, then discount years after year one and note a discount rate of 0% for year one.[25,139,154]

There is no universal discount rate, as it is frequently debated and can vary based on the location of the analysis.[176] Therefore, clearly state the discount rate used and provide the rationale behind the use of that specific rate. For example, the explanation may be that a particular economic evaluation guideline recommends it.[139,154] A discount rate of 3% to 5% is commonly used in base-case analyses.[1,73,77,98] Consider a range of 0% to 10% (or wider) in sensitivity analyses to assess the effect that the discount rate has on the decision.[73,77,98,99,175] Make sure to present both undiscounted and discounted values for costs and outcomes in the results.[73] Use the same discount rate for both measures of costs and outcomes.[77,99]

Inflation

If you use cost data from previous years, you need to adjust for inflation. You may consider using resources (e.g., the Consumer Price Index calculator) to determine the present value.[73,98,214]

Simply put, adjust for inflation for past values and discount future values.

Block 17 – Assumptions

This block is where you state your modeling assumptions.[77] We often do not have the exact data in the population we are interested in evaluating and are basing it off of estimates from data in other populations – where we may not know all the details. As a result, we end up making many assumptions. Assumptions should try to mimic reality as much as possible. Any assumptions made throughout the process on the model structure (how you designed your model or your conceptual framework) and particularly in the analysis of the model must be clearly articulated. It is up to you to evaluate whether the assumptions are reasonable and reflect the realities on the ground. Was it an expert opinion, standard practice, or a specific data source that influenced your decision to make a particular assumption? Be sure to provide the basis for each assumption made, along with the source that may have altered your choice to accept or reject the assumption.

Block 18 – Sensitivity Analysis

Many of the model inputs are often assumptions or "estimates" based on the data we have available, information from expert opinions, or assumptions made by the researchers performing the analysis and may not be precise or cannot be translated entirely to your population of interest.[2,44,53,77,87,99,177] Depending on how and where the data was retrieved, the estimates may greatly fluctuate in terms of quality and accuracy. The estimates may have been compiled from various sources – each with varying methodologies, quality, and differing results for the inputs of interest. For example, one trial estimates a 20% adherence compared to another that states 35% adherence on medication X. This variability in the quality demands assessing the model estimates and assumptions.

Recognizing the limitations of our estimates, determine if the analysis is robust. How do the results change if there are differences in the assumptions or estimates? Is the analysis sensitive to change when input values vary or are adjusted? If one or more of the input values are incorrect, do the results change? Does the decision change? You want to test what will happen to the results if you vary the model inputs. To answer the question, how sensitive is the model to changes in the estimates?[73]

Sensitivity analyses are used to address uncertainty and test the robustness of the model assumptions.[1,2,25,44,53,98,177] They are used to tackle and characterize the uncertainty of the model inputs and must be conducted in any PE analysis.[1,25,44,139] Sensitivity analyses allow you to evaluate all model inputs estimates, assumptions, and test ranges of values for each to determine the impact on the results – the impact on incremental cost and incremental effectiveness – and ultimately the recommendations of the analysis.

Sensitivity analyses help you identify what model inputs or assumptions the analysis is sensitive.[2,29,73,77,139] If the decision or recommendation changes based on a change in input value, the model is sensitive to that particular model input. For example, if you change the discount rate and the decision of which intervention is preferred differs, then the model is sensitive to the discount rate.[29] Evaluate how small or big the changes in the model inputs are and their impact on the results.

The original input estimates we put into the model are part of the base-case.[77,99] We then vary the numbers or input estimates of the base-case using sensitivity analysis. Sensitivity analyses allow you to look at the range that may be evident in the literature and test to see if it impacts the results.[1] Ranges "of plausible values" (best case and worst case) is the range of values where you vary the estimates or model input parameters.[25,73]

- Consider listing all of the parameters where the evidence may not be as strong, or there is room for a wide range of potential values with your team.
- Discuss what may potentially change the results of the analysis as a team and make sure sensitivity analyses are conducted for these parameters.
- For each model input, select an appropriate range (an upper and lower value) that makes the most sense to the situation to be used in the sensitivity analysis.

There is no standard method to determine the range; however, it is recommended to consult experts in the field and review ranges present in the literature.[1,25] Wider ranges are better to use than smaller ranges to demonstrate the robustness of the estimate and model.[1] You may consider re-running the analysis with more narrow ranges if you believe that parameter influences the model.

The most common sensitivity analyses used are deterministic and probabilistic sensitivity analyses.[1,25,73,77,99] **Deterministic sensitivity analyses** evaluate individual parameters and are also referred to as one-way, two-way, and multiple sensitivity analyses. They are used to determine model behavior when model input estimates are varied.[1,77,99]

One-way or univariate sensitivity analyses alter one input variable or estimate at a time and hold all others constant to identify individual estimates' impact on results.[1,2,73] A tornado diagram is an example of a summary of multiple one-way sensitivity analyses and is a great visual representation of the results. The widest bar (shown on the top of a tornado diagram) represents the model estimate with the largest potential effect on the model. As you move down the diagram, the bars of the other estimates become narrower.[1,139,154]

Researchers are expected, at a minimum, to perform at least a one-way sensitivity analysis on crucial individual input estimates. Some researchers may consider a one-way sensitivity analysis on all individual inputs as a starting point.[45]

Two-way and multiple sensitivity analyses are where you simultaneously change at least two variables in the model and evaluate the impact on the results.[1,2,98] If more than one variable is altered at a time, this is called multiple-way sensitivity analysis and is conducted and interpreted in the same fashion as a simple sensitivity analysis.[73]

Probabilistic sensitivity analyses (e.g., Monte Carlo, a simulation) are more analytically complex and entail using mathematical theory and statistics to vary and evaluate all the parameters at once.[1,2,73,77,87,98,99,139,154] An example includes cost-effectiveness acceptability curves, used to present the data visually and incorporate societal WTP thresholds to feature cost-effective interventions.[1,139,15] Other examples include the analysis of extremes and threshold analysis.[73,98]

Regardless of whether you want to change one input or multiple to determine the robustness of the model – make sure you decide which estimates you wish to change and then find the most appropriate sensitivity analyses for that change.

Block 19 – Limitations

State any limitations in the analysis. Transparency is vital. The study limitations and assumptions can limit the generalizability of the analysis. When evaluating the literature, determine whether the limitations were stated and addressed. Examples of limitations include, but not limited to, extrapolating data from short-term studies, questionable quality of the evidence available, specific study designs, databases and sources used, the generalizability of the study results, and actual or potential bias.[1,26,29,177]

Frame 3: Evaluate the Output

Evaluate the Output	**Frame Results** Presentation of the Results (e.g., Title, base case inputs, results, and sensitivity analyses)	**Full Evaluation** What went into the model? What is driving the model? Does it make clinical sense? Where and when can I use this information?
	Frame Discussion, Recommendation and Conclusion Is it generalizable to your situation? What is the recommendation and how will it inform a decision?	

Whether you create it or just read it, you have to evaluate it.

The third and last frame, "Evaluate the Output," is sheds light on the importance of interpreting the data to assess whether the results can be translated and implemented in practice. It also focuses on the art of communicating this science. You will be determining if and how you can use the information generated by the analysis. You will need to reevaluate what is ultimately driving your decisions. An organized, structured approach is critical here to keep it simple and avoid any methodological traps or roadblocks. Make sure to continuously assess the limitations of the analysis and interpret the results with caution.

Block 20 – Frame the Results

This block focuses on the presentation of the results, such as the base case, sensitivity analyses, and others. Here you will be building off and presenting what you have already collected in the other blocks. There are a few things to keep in mind when evaluating and displaying the output.

The manner, content, and the way the results are presented must keep the decision-maker and perspective in mind – that is, it needs to be appropriate for the audience reading the analysis.[25] Determine what is relevant to your audience's perspective. It should answer the decision-maker's question or address a concern. The information presented ultimately impacts the decision-maker.

How easy is it to understand and use the results? Make it simple, easy to interpret, and apply in practice or the real-world.[20] Be deliberate in how you craft and articulate each section. To adequately evaluate the output, it must be presented in a straightforward, transparent, unbiased manner.[25] Transparency and clarity in reporting are essential.[12,139,177] This requires that you understand if and how your data can be used. You need to present enough detail of the methods so that others may either replicate the analysis or at least determine whether it can be generalized to their population of interest.

List all the estimates and parameters used in the study and how they were valued. This list aids in interpreting the results and assessing how easy it is to replicate the analysis.[139,154] Use your data collection form to enter all the input estimates and the data source(s) retrieved for each measure.

Evaluate the quality of the literature that goes into the model and assess the quality of the output. Evaluate each block on the PE Canvas and determine whether the methods and all model inputs used (both costs and outcomes) were appropriate, accurate, and reflect the real-world. Evaluate whether proper statistical methods were used – or determine what statistics to use – and evaluate accordingly.

The format for how you frame the results can depend on whether it is for internal or external publication. An external publication would have to meet the publisher's requirements. The exact style for how you report the results can depend on the institution or journal. Check if any reporting guidelines or instructions are available before submitting the information. Determine to what extent the availability of all the information is essential – especially if you submit an article to a journal with limited space and word count restrictions. The main article should include most (if not all) blocks in the canvas, with priority for additional detail regarding certain elements required by reviewers.[77] Typically, if the analysis is to be submitted to a journal for publication, the general layout is often: abstract, the study or analysis, and additional appendices.

Consider appendices

Results may be included in both the article summarizing the analyses, as well as more detailed technical appendices.[77] When you are restricted with space or word count, consider adding appendices that may be included online for a particular study. Check to see if analyses have online appendices available to evaluate the input and data further.[139,154] Include everything in your full document and then select what you will include in the main paper and what will be in appendices. Journal reviewers may require all documentation at initial submission but will later work with you to determine what to include in the appendices. Thus, be prepared to provide additional information – if required.

Presentation of the Data

One of the most efficient ways to summarize model inputs is through tables that report the values, probabilities, source of the data, and the ranges used to account for uncertainty.[139] The reasons for using specific values, ranges, and data sources are often described in the text of the manuscript or document.

Consider putting the following items in tables:[1,29,44,77,99,139]
- Summary of competing alternatives or interventions.
- Model input estimates or variables – including base case estimates and sensitivity range tested.
- Base case results – including costs, effectiveness, and incremental cost and effectiveness.
- Cost-effectiveness ratios – e.g., average and incremental cost-effectiveness ratios (ICER).
- Secondary analyses, including sensitivity analyses. Be sure also to include the sensitivity analysis ranges used.

Summary of Base Case Results

It is helpful to summarize the results of the model inputs of costs and outcomes into summary measures.[77,139,154] Examples of summary measures based on the type of analysis include: benefit-to-cost ratio for cost-benefit analyses, total costs for cost minimization analyses, cost-effectiveness ratio for CEA, the cost-utility ratio for CUA.[1,44] Report incremental costs and incremental outcome differences between the competing alternatives.[139] Divide the incremental costs by the incremental effectiveness (incremental cost/incremental effectiveness) to obtain the ICER. ICER is the most frequently used, as we are often comparing treatment options or treatment versus no treatment (or doing nothing).[29] An ICER is only reported when the intervention is not dominant or dominated, and when it is relevant for decision-making.[139,154]

If the ICER is negative, that would mean that one strategy is either more costly and less effective (**dominated** strategy, reject this option), and the other strategy is more effective and costs less (**dominant** strategy, accept this option).[1,29,98] A dominant strategy is considered cost-effective. A negative ICER is not calculated or reported, but rather one would either indicate that the strategy was dominant or dominated.[1,21,29,73,98,125]

Consider putting the following items in figures:[29,77]
- Decision tree and/or Markov Model
- Cost-effectiveness plane
- Cost-effectiveness acceptability curve
- Sensitivity or uncertainty analyses

If heterogeneity is present within data and results, consider presenting these in subgroup analyses.[139,154]

Sensitivity Analysis

Clearly state all the assumptions made and which estimates the analysis was sensitive. In other words, clearly explain how or if the results changed with varying assumptions.[77] You can present these using both tables and figures.

Block 21 – Frame the Discussion, Recommendation & Conclusion

This block focuses on summarizing and framing the recommendation(s) and conclusion. Here is where you briefly summarize the results, recommend a specific intervention, or choose a course of action.[29,98]

Determine what is relevant to your audience's perspective and environment (i.e., country-specific, health institution) – this cannot be reiterated enough.[77,99]

Present your recommendation(s) and conclusion in a way that is easy for the ultimate user to understand and apply. Start with the end-user in mind, those who will read and use this information.[28,77,99] Readers or users often have a hard time analyzing and interpreting the data; therefore, recommendations made must be made in a simple, straightforward, and unbiased manner.

The two main questions to answer in this block include:
1. Is it generalizable to your situation?
2. What is the recommendation, and how will it inform a decision?

Determine if the results can be extrapolated or generalizable beyond the study. If so, what are the specific recommendations you would make? If a generalization was made, determine if it was appropriate.[29,86] Are the generalizations and conclusions overstated or exaggerated?[25,29,73] If you are conducting the analysis, avoid these generalizations. Discuss any sensitivity analysis that changed the results of the analysis based on different assumptions and scenarios.[20]

Evaluate how the results impact the decision. The conclusion summarizes how you believe this will inform decision-making. You may not be making a decision based on the results, but the information from these analyses can help shed light on items that may need to be addressed or can be used to better understand each intervention's impact. The decision recommendation(s) generated from these analyses will be perceived as controversial by someone – thus, make sure appropriate rationale is provided to explain why such a proposal is made and its limitations of use.

Block 22 – Full Evaluation and Recap

The analysis should clearly provide a summary of criteria and methods used (all the blocks items used) as well as the model inputs and output (results, discussion, recommendation(s) and conclusion) either in text and/or graphically.[139]

In the full evaluation and recap, you will determine what is relevant to your environment and population.

Start with the title: Clearly state the type of PE analysis conducted – e.g., "Cost-Effectiveness Analysis of ..." to identify the study as an economic evaluation. State the competing alternatives or comparators in the title. You may also consider including a year. Including these items helps with reducing ambiguity and improving identification within databases.[29,139]

The four main questions in the full recap that you will need to answer are:
1. What went into the model?
2. What is driving the model?
3. Does it make clinical sense?
4. Where and when can I use this information?

What went into the model?

Evaluate all model inputs and whether they were appropriately incorporated and measured.[73,177] Assess how the model was set up (model structure and components), the cost and outcome measure used, and how the analysis was conducted and analyzed. Evaluate all the blocks of the canvas and decide whether you can adopt these recommendations based on what went into the model, your situation, or the population. Do the model inputs make sense for your population? How reliable is the data? Did the researchers correct for any bias in the data?[77,99] Make sure the model, analysis, and results are unbiased, believable – and, most importantly – make sense in practice.

Be immensely critical of all components of the analysis. You should evaluate both the quality of the studies that went into the model and the quality of the PE study itself. The quality of the data you put into the model will determine the quality of the output. For example, if patient preferences or quality of life (QOL) measures were used, were the instruments used stated, and are they validated instruments?[73]

What is driving the model?

This question is where you evaluate what you believe is driving the model and the recommendation(s). Generally speaking, what is the idea driving the question from the start? Be clear what model inputs or assumptions are driving the model and what differences affect the results.[20,177] Is a specific input driving the model? Or an intervention strategy? Or specific probabilities or utilities? Sensitivity analysis can help shed light and answer some of these questions. Look to the sensitivity analysis section, and see what input estimates affected the analysis results, and assess whether they make sense.

The results and interpretation of the data can be quite different based on perspective.

Does it make clinical sense?

The competing alternatives and decisions must be realistic. They should address what is actively happening in practice or may occur in the real-world.

Answer the following questions:
- Do the results of the analysis make clinical sense? Is this something you would consider in practice?
- Are the results exaggerated? How much can we "believe"?[25,29]
- Would decision-makers (e.g., clinicians) be willing to recommend or implement this? If not, why?

Where and when can I use this information?

Determine what is relevant to your population and environment – your location and institution.

Answer the following questions:
- Were the generalizations appropriate?[29]
- Can I extrapolate this information?
- How generalizable is this? Is it generalizable to my situation?
- Is it country-specific? Can I adopt their model?
- What are the implications of the information to my institution or population?

Other Considerations

Any sources of funding or non-financial resources used, as well as conflict of interest of the investigators conducting the analyses, should be disclosed.[77,99,139,154]

Pharmacoeconomics Canvas

Define the Criteria

The Question and Objective	Perspective	Competing alternatives *options, interventions or comparators*	Type of Analysis
Patient Population	Location	Time Horizon	Decision Rule or an "Acceptable Threshold"

Frame the Methods then Conduct and/or Evaluate the Analysis

Conceptual Framework
- Design a Conceptual Framework — *Structure the decision question and sequence of events for each alternative*
- Develop an Action Plan
- Design the analytical model
- Design the decision model or study method to be used

The framework and action plan are the basis for the items on the right

Model Inputs

Consequences Model inputs: Appropriate **Outcome Measures** — *Incorporate Probabilities*	Cost Model inputs: Appropriate **Costs**

Resources: Resources available		Evidence and Collection of Data	
Human Resources	Source of data (data source)	Retrieval of Evidence	Data Collection

Adjusting for Time	Assumptions

Sensitivity Analysis	Limitations

Evaluate the Output

Frame Results
Presentation of the Results (e.g., Title, base case inputs, results, and sensitivity analyses)

Full Evaluation
- What went into the model?
- What is driving the model?
- Does it make clinical sense?
- Where and when can I use this information?

Frame Discussion, Recommendation and Conclusion
- Is it generalizable to your situation?
- What is the recommendation and how will it inform a decision?

Up Next

In this chapter, we discussed the standards and approaches to conduct and evaluate PE analyses. The PE Canvas was introduced and explained in detail, including the statement of its use. In the next section, you will find the abbreviations and resources used throughout the book.

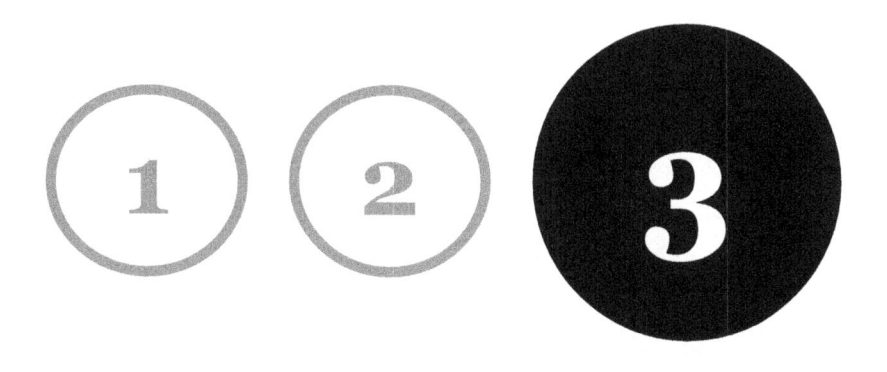

SECTION 3: PUTTING IT ALL TOGETHER

Brief Summary of the Book

Let's quickly recap

In summary, pharmacoeconomics (PE) is a type of outcomes research and a subset of health economics that focuses on pharmaceutical interventions.[1,29,53] PE is used to inform resource allocation decisions and define effective pharmaceutical policies.[1,25,29,53,73,88] PE analyses are only one tool in healthcare decision-making. Several other factors are integrated into the decision-making process.

Decide what goes into your decision criteria. No single assessment, checklist, or guidelines will work for every decision question. When performing economic analyses, the general process includes using the evidence we have to fill in the model, making assumptions, and then accounting for uncertainty.

There are several limitations to the process; therefore, it is crucial to interpret the results with caution. You may not be making a decision based on the results of PE analyses, but the information provided from these analyses can help shed light on items that may need to be addressed or can be used as a way to better understand each intervention's impact. Whether you create it or just read PE analyses, you have to evaluate it.

Learning the art of pharmacoeconomics in the manner addressed in the book will help tell stories of impact through a more objective and evidence-based approach. The hope is that it will enable the information that is generated to be more useful in practice. Use the material in this book to map out a master plan.

The field of OR is continuously growing. There is a need for health professionals to be at the forefront of identifying and implementing multidisciplinary interventions and programs of quality and assessing the impact of healthcare interventions on the patient care experience.[79] More research is needed to identify policies that increase access, reduce costs, and improve health outcomes.

Section 1 provided summaries on the topics of healthcare resource allocation, value, decision-making, and the different types of economic analyses. The decisions made at an institution-level can have ripple effects and impact populations. Our impact can start from our institutions and expand to the global communities. Innovation travels. An overarching goal should be to provide more objective, evidence-based decision-making in healthcare – with the ultimate goal of adding value. Value embodies a broad collection of factors and experiences relevant to and utilized by individuals, institutions, and society.

The significance of surrounding yourself with the "right" people cannot be understated. Just as you would create a team before building or incorporating a product or service, the same applies to build a great team to conduct this type of research. Section 2 answered common questions concerning teams in PE analyses. The strength of a team is in the skills and perspectives each member provides. Seek new ways to partner with diverse professionals, and do not forget to use design thinking. Tools created in this book – such as the lifecycle of a PE analysis, PE base, domains, the elements of The Process, and the PE Canvas – will be useful as you begin the journey of conducting or evaluating PE analyses. Consider using the PE Canvas in addition to other decision-making tools or strategies. The various checklists, guidance, and strategies are continuously updated; therefore, it is advised that you always check for the latest recommendations as you conduct or evaluate PE analyses. Remember, researchers are designers, and designers are researchers. You are a designer – all you need is to get started!

Abbreviations

AHRQ	Agency for Healthcare Research and Quality
AMCP	Academy of Managed Care Pharmacy
APN	Advanced Practice Nurses
CBA	cost-benefit analysis
CCA	cost-consequence analysis
CE	cost-effective or cost-effectiveness
CEA	cost-effectiveness analysis
CER	comparative effectiveness research
CHEERS	Consolidated Health Economic Evaluation Reporting Standards
CMS	Centers for Medicare and Medicaid Services
COI	cost-of-illness
CUA	cost-utility analysis
DDS	Doctor of Dental Surgery
DSAEK	descemet stripping automated endothelial keratoplasty
DMD	Doctor of Medicine in Dentistry
DO	Doctor of Osteopathic Medicine
EBM	evidence-based medicine
ECHO	Economic, Clinical, and Humanistic Outcomes
EQLS	European Quality of Life Index
EQ-5D	EuroQol 5D
e.g.	for example
EHR	electronic health records
EMR	electronic medical records
FCBT	face-to-face cognitive behavioral therapy
FDA	Food and Drug Administration
GDP	gross domestic product
HEOR	health economics and outcomes research
HIO	healthcare – innovation – outcomes
HRQOL	health-related quality of life
ICBT	internet-based cognitive behavioral therapy

ICER	incremental cost-effectiveness ratio
ICUR	incremental cost-utility ratio
i.e.	as in
IRB	institutional review board
ISPOR	Professional Society for Health Economics and Outcomes Research
MALDI-TOF	Matrix- assisted laser desorption ionization-time of flight
MD	Doctor of Medicine
NCQA	National Committee for Quality Assurance
NB	net benefit
NP	nurse practitioners
NPC	National Pharmaceutical Council
QALY	quality-adjusted life year
QWB	Quality of Well-Being Scale
OR	outcomes research
PA	physician assistant
PBM	pharmacy benefits management
PE	pharmacoeconomics
PEOR	pharmacoeconomics and outcomes research
PharmD	Doctor of Pharmacy
PK	penetrating keratoplasty
PSA	prostate-specific antigen
PT	physical therapist
P&T	pharmacy and therapeutics
QALY	quality adjusted life years
QOL	quality of life
RCT	randomized controlled trial
RN	registered nurse
RPh	registered pharmacist
RWD	real-world data
RWE	real-world evidence
SF-36	Short-form 36
US	United States
VP	value proposition
vs.	versus
YHL	Years of Health Life

Abbreviations

WHO   World Health Organization
WTP   willingness-to-pay
Δ   incremental

References

1. Mackinnon GE. Understanding Health Outcomes and Pharmacoeconomics. 2013. Jones &. Bartlett Learning, LLC and Ascend Learning Company.
2. Edlin R, McCabe, Hulme C, Hall P, et al Cost-Effectiveness Modeling for Health Technology Assessment: A Practical Course. 2015. ADIS.
3. Bendavid E, Duong A, Sagan C, et al. Health Aid Is Allocated Efficiently, But Not Optimally: Insights From A Review Of Cost-Effectiveness Studies. Health Aff (Millwood). 2015 Jul;34(7):1188-95.
4. Persad G, Wertheimer A, Emanuel EJ. Principles for allocation of scarce medical interventions. Lancet. 2009 Jan 31;373(9661):423-31.
5. Edwards RT, Charles JM, Lloyd-Williams H. Public health economics: a systematic review of guidance for the economic evaluation of public health interventions and discussion of key methodological issues. BMC Public Health. 2013 Oct 24;13:1001.
6. Singer P, Why we ration healthcare. The New York Times. July 19, 2009. Available at: https://www.nytimes.com/2009/07/19/magazine/19healthcare-t.html
7. Professional Society for Health Economics and Outcomes Research (ISPOR). ISPOR 2020 Top 10 HEOR Trends. Available at: https://www.ispor.org/docs/default-source/heor-resources/2020-top-10-heor-trends_v-online_00120191219.pdf?sfvrsn=9eebcb74_0
8. Modic MT, Lasalvia L, Merges R. Standardization and personalization: lessons from other industries. Siemens Healthineers Insights series. Issue 6. Available at: https://www.siemens-healthineers.com/en-us/insights/news/standardization-personalization-other-industries.html
9. Sanders GD, Maciejewski ML, Basu A. Overview of Cost-effectiveness Analysis. JAMA. 2019 Apr 9;321(14):1400-1401.
10. Shrank WH. The evolving role of health services researchers in a transforming healthcare system. Healthc (Amst). 2013 Dec;1(3-4):61-2.
11. Burkholder R, Dougherty JS, Neves LA. ISPOR's Initiative on US Value Assessment Frameworks: An Industry Perspective. Value Health. 2018 Feb;21(2):173-175.
12. Food and Drug Administration (FDA). Drug and Device Manufacturer Communications With Payors, Formulary Committees, and Similar Entities – Questions and Answers Guidance for Industry and Review Staff. June 2018. Available at: https://www.fda.gov/regulatory-information/search-fda-guidance-documents/drug-and-device-manufacturer-communications-payors-formulary-committees-and-similar-entities
13. Vermeulen LC, Eddington ND, Gourdine MA, et al. ASHP Foundation Pharmacy Forecast 2019: Strategic Planning Advice for Pharmacy Departments in Hospitals and Health Systems. Am J Health Syst Pharm. 2019 Jan 16;76(2):71-100.
14. Buxbaum JD, John N, Mafi JN, et al. Tackling Low-Value Care: A New "Top Five" for Purchaser Action. Health Affairs Blog. Nov 2017. Available at: https://www.healthaffairs.org/do/10.1377/hblog20171117.664355/full/
15. Mafi JN, Russell K, Bortz BA, et al. Low-Cost, High-Volume Health Services Contribute The Most To Unnecessary Health Spending. Health Aff (Millwood). 2017 Oct 1;36(10):1701-1704.

References

16. VBID Health. The Top Five Low-Value Services. Available at: http://www.vbidhealth.com/low-value-care-top-five-services.php
17. Center for Value-Based Insurance Design (V-BID). V-BID X Infographic. Available at: https://vbidcenter.org/wp-content/uploads/2019/03/V-BID-X-Infographic-030919.pdf
18. Neumann PJ, Weissman H. The FDA's New Guidance On Payer Communications: Implications For Real-World Data And Value-Based Contracts. Nov 2018. Available at: https://www.healthaffairs.org/do/10.1377/hblog20180712.816686/full/
19. National Pharmaceutical Council. Thinking Differently About How We Assess Health Value: Policy Experts Clash Over Budget Impact Assessments at ISPOR. Available at: https://www.npcnow.org/newsroom/commentary/thinking-differently-about-how-we-assess-health-value
20. National Pharmaceutical Council. Guiding Practices for Patient-Centered Value Assessment. Available at: https://www.npcnow.org/guidingpractices
21. Garrison LP Jr, Kamal-Bahl S, Towse A. Toward a Broader Concept of Value: Identifying and Defining Elements for an Expanded Cost-Effectiveness Analysis. Value Health. 2017 Feb;20(2):213-216.
22. Center for Value-Based Insurance Design (V-BID). V-BID Infographic. Mar 2020. Available at: https://vbidcenter.org/wp-content/uploads/2016/02/V-BID-Update-3.2.20.pdf
23. Center for Value-Based Insurance Design (V-BID). V-BID and Diabetes Infographic. Aug 2019. Available at: https://vbidcenter.org/wp-content/uploads/2018/09/V-BID-and-Diabetes-Info-8.26.2019.pdf
24. Center for Value-Based Insurance Design (V-BID). V-BID Financial Impact Infographic. Aug 2019. Available at: https://vbidcenter.org/wp-content/uploads/2017/10/Financial-Impact-of-V-BID-8.28.2019.pdf
25. Malone PM, Malone MJ, Park SK. Drug Information A guide for pharmacist. 2018. McGraw-Hill Education.
26. Birnbaum HG, Greenberg PE. Decision Making in a world of comparative effectiveness research. 2017. ADIS.
27. Kaakeh R, Kaakeh A. Does Your Behaviour Add Value? Applying Metrics Can Help. Forbes Middle East. May 2018. Available at: https://www.forbesmiddleeast.com/innovation/opinion/does-your-behaviour-add-value-applying-metrics-can-help
28. Padula WV, McQueen RB, Pronovost PJ. Can Economic Model Transparency Improve Provider Interpretation of Cost-effectiveness Analysis? Evaluating Tradeoffs Presented by the Second Panel on Cost-Effectiveness in Health and Medicine. Med Care. 2017 Nov; 55(11):909-911
29. Rascati KL. Essentials of Pharmacoeconomics. 2014. Lippincott Williams & Wilkins, a Wolters Kluwer business.
30. Schumock Gt, Stubbings J, Wiest MD, et al. National trends in prescription drug expenditures and projects for 2018. Am J Health Syst Pharm. 2018 Jul 15; 75(14):1023-1038
31. The PEW Charitable Trusts. A Look at Drug Spending in the U.S. Feb 27 2018. Available at: https://www.pewtrusts.org/en/research-and-analysis/fact-sheets/2018/02/a-look-at-drug-spending-in-the-us
32. Centers for Medicaid and Medicare Services. National Health Expenditures 2018 Highlights. Updated Dec 2019. Available at: https://www.cms.gov/files/document/highlights.pdf
33. Yu NL, Atteberry P, Bach PB. Spending on Prescription Drugs in the US: Where does all the money go? Health Affairs Blog. July 2018. Available at: https://www.healthaffairs.org/do/10.1377/hblog20180726.670593/full/
34. Centers for Disease Control and Prevention. Health Expenditures. 2017. Available at: https://www.cdc.gov/nchs/fastats/health-expenditures.htm

35. Papanicolas I, Woskie LR, Jha A. Health care spending in the United States and other high-income countries. The Commonwealth Fund. Available at: https://www.commonwealthfund.org/publications/journal-article/2018/mar/health-care-spending-united-states-and-other-high-income
36. Schumock GT, Stubbings J, Hoffman JM, et al. National trends in prescription drug expenditures and projections for 2019. Am J Health Syst Pharm. 2019 Jul 18;76(15):1105-1121.
37. United Nations Department of Economic and Social Affairs. World Economic Situation and Prospects. Jan 2019. Available at: https://www.un.org/development/desa/publications/publication/world-economic-situation-and-prospects-2019
38. World Health Organization (WHO). WHO Constitution. Available at: https://www.who.int/about/who-we-are/constitution
39. Remme M, Martinez-Alvarez M, Vassall A. Cost-Effectiveness Thresholds in Global Health: Taking a Multisectoral Perspective. Value Health. 2017 Apr;20(4):699-704.
40. Neumann PJ, Willke RJ, Garrison LP Jr. A Health Economics Approach to US Value Assessment Frameworks-Introduction: An ISPOR Special Task Force Report [1]. Value Health. 2018 Feb; 21(2):119-123
41. Garrison LP Jr, Pauly MV, Willke RJ, et al. An Overview of Value, Perspective, and Decision Context- A Health Economics Approach: An ISPOR Special Task Force Report [2]. Value Health. 2018 Feb;21(2):124-130.
42. Garrison LP Jr, Neumann PJ, Willke RJ, et al. A Health Economics Approach to US Value Assessment Frameworks - Summary and Recommendations of the ISPOR Special Task Force Report [7]. Value Health. 2018 Feb; 21(2):161-165
43. Asche CV. Applying Comparative Effectiveness Data to Medical Decision Making: A Practical Guide. 2016. ADIS.
44. Arnold RJ. Pharmacoeconomics: From Theory to Practice. 2010. Taylor and Francis Group, LLC.
45. Willke RJ, Neumann PJ, Garrison LP Jr, et al. Review of Recent US Value Frameworks-A Health Economics Approach: An ISPOR Special Task Force Report [6]. Value Health. 2018 Feb;21(2):155-160.
46. Perfetto EM, Oehrlein EM, Boutin M, et al. Value to whom? The patient voice in the value discussion. Value Health 2017;20:286–91.
47. Goetghebeur MM, Wagner M, Khoury H, et al. Evidence and Value: Impact on DEcisionMaking--the EVIDEM framework and potential applications. BMC Health Serv Res. 2008 Dec 22;8:270.
48. Perfetto EM. ISPOR's Initiative on US Value Assessment Frameworks: A Missed Opportunity for ISPOR and Patients. Value Health. 2018 Feb;21(2):169-170.
49. Garrison LP Jr, Kamal-Bahl S, Towse A. Toward a Broader Concept of Value: Identifying and Defining Elements for an Expanded Cost-Effectiveness Analysis. Value Health. 2017 Feb;20(2):213-216.
50. Kaakeh R. 5 Strategies to Incorporate on the Path to Creating Value in Public Health. The Pursuit. August 2018. Available at: https://sph.umich.edu/pursuit/2018posts/create-value-in-public-health.html
51. Horn SD, Gassaway J. Practice based evidence: incorporating clinical heterogeneity and patient-reported outcomes for comparative effectiveness research. Med Care. 2010 Jun;48(6 Suppl):S17-22.
52. Sculpher M. ISPOR's Initiative on US Value Assessment Frameworks: Seeking a Role for Health Economics. Value Health. 2018 Feb;21(2):171-172.
53. Pradelli L, Wertheimer A. Pharmacoeconomics: Principles and Practice. 2012. SEEd.
54. World Health Organization (WHO). WHO updates global guidance on medicines and diagnostic tests to address health challenges, prioritize highly effective therapeutics, and improve affordable access. News Release. July 2019. Available at: https://www.who.int/news-room/detail/09-07-2019-who-updates-

References

global-guidance-on-medicines-and-diagnostic-tests-to-address-health-challenges-prioritize-highly-effective-therapeutics-and-improve-affordable-access

55. National Pharmaceutical Council. Thinking Differently About How We Assess Health Value; Current Landscape: Value Assessment Frameworks. Mar 2016. Available at: https://www.npcnow.org/publication/current-landscape-value-assessment-frameworks
56. Neumann PJ, Willke RJ, Garrison LP Jr. A Health Economics Approach to US Value Assessment Frameworks - Introduction: An ISPOR Special Task Force Report [1]. Value Health. 2018 Feb; 21(2):119-123
57. Solow B, Pezalla EJ. ISPOR's Initiative on US Value Assessment Frameworks: The Use of Cost-Effectiveness Research in Decision Making among US Insurers. Value Health. 2018 Feb;21(2):166-168.
58. Schnipper LE, Davidson HE, Wollins DS, et al. Updating the American Society of Clinical Oncology value framework: revisions and reflections in response to comments received. J Clin Oncol 2016;34:2925–34.
59. Vermeulen LC, Kolesar J, Crismon ML, et al. ASHP Foundation Pharmacy Forecast 2018: Strategic Planning Advice for Pharmacy Departments in Hospitals and Health Systems. Am J Health Syst Pharm. 2018 Jan 15;75(2):23-54.
60. Phelps CE, Lakdawalla DN, Basu A, et al. Approaches to Aggregation and Decision Making – A Health Economics Approach: An ISPOR Special Task Force Report [5]. Value Health. 2018 Feb;21(2):146-154.
61. Thokala P, Devlin N, Marsh K, et al. Multiple Criteria Decision Analysis for Health Care Decision Making--An Introduction: Report 1 of the ISPOR MCDA Emerging Good Practices Task Force. Value Health. 2016 Jan;19(1):1-13.
62. Academy of Managed Care Pharmacy. The Academy of Managed Care Pharmacy's Concepts in Managed Care Pharmacy Outcomes Research. April 2012. Available at: https://www.amcp.org/sites/default/files/2019-03/Outcomes%20Research%204.2012.pdf
63. Schumock GT, Walton SM, Park HY, et al. Factors that influence prescribing decisions. Ann Pharmacother. 2004 Apr;38(4):557-62.
64. Cheema E, Alhomoud FK, Kinsara ASA, et al. The impact of pharmacists-led medicines reconciliation on healthcare outcomes in secondary care: A systematic review and meta-analysis of randomized controlled trials. PLoS One. 2018;13(3):e0193510.
65. Hazen ACM, de Bont AA, Boelman L, et al. The degree of integration of non-dispensing pharmacists in primary care practice and the impact on health outcomes: A systematic review. Res Social Adm Pharm. 2018 Mar;14(3):228-240.
66. Garrison LP Jr, Neumann PJ, Erickson P, et al. Using real-world data for coverage and payment decisions: the ISPOR Real-World Data Task Force report. Value Health. 2007 Sep-Oct;10(5):326-35.
67. Schumock, GT, Meek PD, Ploetz PA, et al. Economic evaluations of clinical pharmacy services-1988-1995. Pharmacotherapy. 1996; 16(6): 1188-1208
68. Schumock GT, Butler MG, Meek PD, et al. Evidence of the economic benefit of clinical pharmacy services: 1996-2000. Pharmacotherapy. 2003; 23(1): 113-132
69. Perez A, Doloresco F, Hoffman JM, et al. Economic evaluations of clinical pharmacy services: 2001-2005. Pharmacotherapy. 2008: 28 (11): 285e-323e
70. Chisholm-Burns MA, Graff Zivin JS, Lee JK, et al. Economic effects of pharmacists on health outcomes in the United States: A systematic review. Am J Health Syst Pharm. 2010 Oct 1;67(19):1624-34
71. Chisholm-Burn MA, Lee JK, Spivey CA, et al. US pharmacists' effect as team members on patient care systematic review and meta-analyses. Med Care, 2010; 48: 923-933
72. Touchette DR, Doloresco F, Suda KJ, et al. Economic evaluations of clinical pharmacy services: 2006-2010. Pharmacotherapy. 2014 Aug;34(8):771-93.

73. McCarthy RL, Schafermeyer KW, Plake KS. Introduction to Healthcare Delivery A Primer for Pharmacists. 2012. Jones & Bartlett Learning, LLC.
74. Academy of Managed Care Pharmacy. Outcomes Research. Feb 2015. https://www.amcp.org/about/managed-care-pharmacy-101/managed-care-pharmacy-power-point-presentations
75. Laxminarayan R, Chow J, Shahid-Salles SA. Intervention Cost-Effectiveness: Overview of Main Messages. In: Jamison DT, Breman JG, Measham AR, et al., editors. Disease Control Priorities in Developing Countries. 2nd edition. Washington (DC): The International Bank for Reconstruction and Development / The World Bank; 2006. Chapter 2. Co-published by Oxford University Press, New York.
76. Cookson R, Mirelman AJ, Griffin S, et al. Using Cost-Effectiveness Analysis to Address Health Equity Concerns. Value Health. 2017 Feb;20(2):206-212.
77. Sanders GD, Neumann PJ, Basu A, et al. Recommendations for Conduct, Methodological Practices, and Reporting of Cost-effectiveness Analyses: Second Panel on Cost-Effectiveness in Health and Medicine. JAMA. 2016 Sep 13; 316(10):1093-103
78. Husereau D, Drummond M, Petrou S, et al. ISPOR Health Economic Evaluation Publication Guidelines - CHEERS Good Reporting Practices Task Force. Consolidated Health Economic Evaluation Reporting Standards (CHEERS) — explanation and elaboration: a report of the ISPOR Health Economic Evaluation Publication Guidelines Good Reporting Practices Task Force. Value Health. 2013 Mar-Apr; 16(2):231-50
79. Foundation for Health Services Research. Health Outcomes Research: A Primer. 1994. Available at: https://studylib.net/doc/11579500/health-outcomes-research--a-primer
80. Academy of Managed Care Pharmacy. Outcomes Research. July 2019. Available at: https://www.amcp.org/about/managed-care-pharmacy-101/concepts-managed-care-pharmacy/outcomes-research
81. Drummond M, Brown R, Fendrick AM, et al. Use of pharmacoeconomics information--report of the ISPOR Task Force on use of pharmacoeconomic/health economic information in health-care decision making. Value Health. 2003 Jul-Aug;6(4):407-16.
82. Gassman AL, Nguyen CP, Joffe HV. FDA Regulation of Prescription Drugs. N Engl J Med. 2017 Feb 16;376(7):674-682.
83. Frieden TR. Evidence for Health Decision Making — Beyond Randomized, Controlled Trials. Aug 2017. N Engl J Med 2017; 377:465-475
84. Outcomes Research: Fact Sheet. March 2000. Agency for Healthcare Research and Quality, Rockville, MD. Available at: http://archive.ahrq.gov/research/findings/factsheets/outcomes/outfact/outcomes-and-research.html
85. Academy of Managed Care Pharmacy. The Academy of Managed Care Pharmacy's Concepts in Managed Care Pharmacy Outcomes Research. April 2012. Available at: https://www.amcp.org/sites/default/files/2019-03/Outcomes%20Research%204.2012.pdf
86. Zhang F, He X, Xiang W, et al. Assessment of the quality of pharmacoeconomic evaluation literature in China. J Med Econ. 2017 May;20(5):510-517
87. Wang Z, Salmon JW, Walton SM. Cost-effectiveness analysis and the formulary decision-making process. J Manag Care Pharm. 2004 Jan-Feb;10(1):48-59.
88. Hutubessy R, Chisholm D, Edejer TT. Generalized cost-effectiveness analysis for national-level priority-setting in the health sector. Cost Eff Resour Alloc. 2003 Dec 19;1(1):8.
89. Kaboli PJ, Hoth AB, McClimon BJ, et al. Clinical pharmacists and inpatient medical care: systematic review. Arch Intern Med. 2006; 166:955-964
90. Pickard AS, Hung SY. An update on evidence of clinical pharmacy services' impact on health related quality of life. Ann Pharmacother. 2006 Sep;40(9):1623-34.

References

91. Nkansah N, Mostovetsky O, Yu C, et al. Effect of outpatient pharmacists' non-dispensing roles on patient outcomes and prescribing patterns. Cochrane Database of Systematic Reviews. 2010; Jul 7;(7):CD000336.
92. Kozma CM, Reeder CE, Schulz RM. Economic, clinical, and humanistic outcomes: a planning model for pharmacoeconomic research. Clin Ther. 1993 Nov-Dec;15(6):1121-32; discussion 1120.
93. Food and Drug Administration (FDA). Real World Evidence. May 2019. Available at: https://www.fda.gov/science-research/science-and-research-special-topics/real-world-evidence
94. Professional Society for Health Economics and Outcomes Research (ISPOR). Real-World Evidence. July 2018. Available at: https://www.ispor.org/ strategic-initiatives/real-world-evidence.
95. Food and Drug Administration (FDA). Drug and Device Manufacturer Communications With Payors, Formulary Committees, and Similar Entities – Questions and Answers Guidance for Industry and Review Staff. June 2018. Available at: https://www.fda.gov/regulatory-information/search-fda-guidance-documents/drug-and-device-manufacturer-communications-payors-formulary-committees-and-similar-entities
96. Food and Drug Administration (FDA). Real World Evidence. May 2019. Available at: https://www.fda.gov/science-research/science-and-research-special-topics/real-world-evidence
97. Agency for Healthcare Research and Quality (AHRQ). AHRQ Comparative Effectiveness Technical Briefs [Internet]. Rockville (MD): Agency for Healthcare Research and Quality (US); 2009-. Available at: https://www.ncbi.nlm.nih.gov/books/NBK242351/
98. Muenning P. Designing and conducting cost-effectiveness analyses in medicine and healthcare. San Francisco: Josey-Bass, 2002
99. Sanders GD, Neumann PJ, Basu A, et al. Recommendations for conduct, methodological practices, and reporting of cost-effectiveness analyses: Second Panel on Cost-Effectiveness in Health and Medicine. JAMA. 2016. eAppendix.
100. Arnold RJ. Pharmacoeconomics: From Theory to Practice. 2010. Taylor and Francis Group, LLC.
101. Levy J, Rosenberg M, Vanness D. A Transparent and Consistent Approach to Assess US Outpatient Drug Costs for Use in Cost-Effectiveness Analyses. Value Health. 2018 Jun;21(6):677-684.
102. Rothwell PM. External validity of randomised controlled trials: "to whom do the results of this trial apply?" Lancet. 2005 Jan 1-7;365(9453):82-93.
103. Yuan H, Ali MS, Brouwer ES, et al. Real-World Evidence: What It Is and What It Can Tell Us According to the International Society for Pharmacoepidemiology (ISPE) Comparative Effectiveness Research (CER) Special Interest Group (SIG). Clin Pharmacol Ther. 2018 Aug;104(2):239-241.
104. Sherman RE, Anderson SA, Dal Pan GJ, et al. Real-World Evidence - What Is It and What Can It Tell Us?. N Engl J Med. 2016 Dec 8;375(23):2293-2297.
105. Revicki DA, Frank L. Pharmacoeconomic evaluation in the real world. Effectiveness versus efficacy studies. Pharmacoeconomics. 1999 May;15(5):423-34.
106. Ghaibi S, Ipema H, Gabay M; American Society of Health System Pharmacists. ASHP guidelines on the pharmacist's role in providing drug information. Am J Health Syst Pharm. 2015 Apr 1;72(7):573-7.
107. Ramsey SD, Willke RJ, Glick H, et al. Cost-effectiveness analysis alongside clinical trials II-An ISPOR Good Research Practices Task Force report. Value Health. 2015 Mar;18(2):161-72.
108. Malone DC, Brown M, Hurwitz JT, et al. Real-World Evidence: Useful in the Real World of US Payer Decision Making? How? When? And What Studies? Value Health. 2018 Mar;21(3):326-333. doi: 10.1016/j.jval.2017.08.3013. Epub 2017 Oct 18.
109. Food and Drug Administration (FDA). Framework for FDA's Real-World Evidence Program. Dec 2018. Available at: https://www.fda.gov/media/120060/download

110. Food and Drug Administration (FDA). Submitting Documents Using Real-World Data and Real-World Evidence to FDA for Drugs and Biologics Guidance for Industry. May 2019. Available at: https://www.fda.gov/regulatory-information/search-fda-guidance-documents/submitting-documents-using-real-world-data-and-real-world-evidence-fda-drugs-and-biologics-guidance
111. Food and Drug Administration (FDA). Use of Real-World Evidence to Support Regulatory Decision-Making for Medical Devices. Aug 2017. Available at: https://www.fda.gov/regulatory-information/search-fda-guidance-documents/use-real-world-evidence-support-regulatory-decision-making-medical-device. https://www.fda.gov/media/99447/download
112. Bryant PJ, Pace HA. The Pharmacist's Guide to Evidence-Based Medicine for Clinical Decision-making. 2014. American Society of Health-System Pharmacists.
113. Berger ML, Sox H, Willke RJ, et al. Good Practices for Real-World Data Studies of Treatment and/or Comparative Effectiveness: Recommendations from the Joint ISPOR-ISPE Special Task Force on Real-World Evidence in Health Care Decision Making. Value Health. 2017 Sep;20(8):1003-1008.
114. Jones LK, Pulk R, Gionfriddo MR, et al. Utilizing big data to provide better health at lower cost. Am J Health Syst Pharm. 2018 Apr 1;75(7):427-435.
115. Cave A, Kurz X, Arlett P. Real-world data for regulatory decision making: challenges and possible solutions for Europe. Clin Pharm Ther. 2019;106(1).
116. Livet M, Haines ST, Curran GM, et al. Implementation Science to Advance Care Delivery: A Primer for Pharmacists and Other Health Professionals. Pharmacotherapy. 2018 May;38(5):490-502.
117. Brown CH, Curran G, Palinkas LA, et al. An Overview of Research and Evaluation Designs for Dissemination and Implementation. Annu Rev Public Health. 2017 Mar 20;38:1-22
118. Hall R, Lieberman M. Economics Principles & Applications, 5th ed. 2010. South-Western, Cengage Learning.
119. Drummond MF, Sculpher MJ, Torrance G, et al. Methods for the Economic Evaluation of Health Care Programmes. (3rd ed.). 2005. New York: Oxford University Press
120. Professional Society for Health Economics and Outcomes Research (ISPOR). ISPOR Good Practices for Outcomes Research. Available at: https://www.ispor.org/heor-resources/good-practices-for-outcomes-research
121. Suh DC, Okpara IR, Agnese WB, et al. Application of pharmacoeconomics to formulary decision making in managed care organizations. Am J Manag Care. 2002 Feb;8(2):161-9. Review.
122. Jena AB, Philipson T. Cost-effectiveness as a price control. Health Aff (Millwood). 2007 May-Jun;26(3):696-703.
123. Anagnostis E, Wordell C, Guharoy R, et al. A national survey on hospital formulary management processes. J Pharm Pract. 2011 Aug;24(4):409-16
124. Tordoff JM, Murphy JE, Norris PT, et al. Use of centrally developed pharmacoeconomic assessments for local formulary decisions. Am J Health Syst Pharm. 2006 Sep 1;63(17):1613-8
125. Carias C, Chesson HW, Grosse SD, et al. Recommendations of the Second Panel on Cost Effectiveness in Health and Medicine: A Reference, Not a Rule Book. Am J Prev Med. 2018 Apr;54(4):600-602.
126. Shrank WH, Fox SA, Kirk A, et al. The effect of pharmacy benefit design on patient-physician communication about costs. J Gen Intern Med. 2006 Apr;21(4):334-9.
127. Academy of Managed Care Pharmacy. Outcomes Research. July 2019. Available at: https://www.amcp.org/about/managed-care-pharmacy-101/concepts-managed-care-pharmacy/outcomes-research

References

128. Sanders GD, Neumann PJ, Basu A, et al. Recommendations for Conduct, Methodological Practices, and Reporting of Cost-effectiveness Analyses: Second Panel on Cost-Effectiveness in Health and Medicine. JAMA. 2016 Sep 13;316(10):1093-103.
129. Professional Society for Health Economics and Outcomes Research (ISPOR). ISPOR Good Practices for Outcomes Research. Available at: https://www.ispor.org/heor-resources/good-practices-for-outcomes-research
130. Professional Society for Health Economics and Outcomes Research (ISPOR). ISPOR: Pharmacoeconomic Guidelines Around The World. Available at: https://tools.ispor.org/peguidelines/
131. Garber AM, Sox HC. The role of costs in comparative effectiveness research. Health Aff (Millwood). 2010 Oct;29(10):1805-11.
132. National Institute for Health and Care Excellence. NICE explores extending its use of data to inform its guidance. June 2019. Available at: https://www.nice.org.uk/news/article/nice-explores-extending-its-use-of-data-to-inform-its-guidance.
133. Professional Society for Health Economics and Outcomes Research (ISPOR). ISPOR Good Practices for Outcomes Research. Available at: https://www.ispor.org/heor-resources/good-practices-for-outcomes-research
134. Hill SR, Mitchell AS, Henry DA. Problems with the interpretation of pharmacoeconomic analyses: a review of submissions to the Australian Pharmaceutical Benefits Scheme. JAMA. 2000 Apr 26;283(16):2116-21.
135. Luce BR. What will it take to make cost-effectiveness analysis acceptable in the United States? Med Care. 2005 Jul;43(7 Suppl):44-8.
136. Neumann PJ. Why don't Americans use cost-effectiveness analysis? Am J Manag Care. 2004 May;10(5):308-12.
137. Watson SI, Sahota H, Taylor CA, et al. Cost-effectiveness of health care service delivery interventions in low- and middle-income countries: a systematic review. Glob Health Res Policy. 2018;3:17.
138. Brooke BS, Kaji AH, Itani KMF. Practical Guide to Cost-effectiveness Analysis. JAMA Surg. 2020 Jan 29.
139. Husereau D, Drummond M, Petrou S, et al. CHEERS Task Force. Consolidated Health Economic Evaluation Reporting Standards (CHEERS) statement. Value Health. 2013 Mar-Apr;16(2):e1-5.
140. Makhinova T, Rascati K. Pharmacoeconomics education in US colleges and schools of pharmacy. Am J Pharm Educ. 2013 Sep 12;77(7):145.
141. Cavanaugh TM, Buring S, Cluxton R. A pharmacoeconomics and formulary management collaborative project to teach decision analysis principles. Am J Pharm Educ. 2012 Aug 10;76(6):115.
142. Soliman AM, Hussein M, Abdulhalim AM. Pharmacoeconomic education in Egyptian schools of pharmacy. Am J Pharm Educ. 2013 Apr 12;77(3):57.
143. Kane-Gill S, Reddy P, Gupta SR, et al. Guidelines for pharmacoeconomic and outcomes research fellowship training programs: joint guidelines from the American college of clinical pharmacy and the international society of pharmacoeconomics and outcomes research. Pharmacotherapy. 2008 Dec;28(12):1552.
144. Rascati KL, Drummond MF, Annemans L, et al. Education in pharmacoeconomics: an international multidisciplinary view. Pharmacoeconomics. 2004;22(3):139-47.
145. Ozaki AF, Nakagawa S, Jackevicius CA. Cross-cultural Comparison of Pharmacy Students' Attitudes, Knowledge, Practice, and Barriers Regarding Evidence-based Medicine. Am J Pharm Educ. 2019 Jun;83(5):6710.

146. Perez A, Rabionet S, Bleidt B. Teaching Research Skills to Student Pharmacists in One Semester: An Applied Research Elective. Am J Pharm Educ. 2017 Feb 25;81(1):16.
147. Law AV, Jackevicius CA, Bounthavong M. A monograph assignment as an integrative application of evidence-based medicine and pharmacoeconomic principles. Am J Pharm Educ. 2011 Feb 10;75(1):1.
148. Reddy M, Rascati K, Wahawisan J, et al. Pharmacoeconomic education in US colleges and schools of pharmacy: an update. Am J Pharm Educ. 2008 Jun 15;72(3):51.
149. Slejko JF, Libby AM, Nair KV, et al. Pharmacoeconomics and outcomes research degree-granting PhD programs in the United States. Res Social Adm Pharm. 2013 Jan-Feb;9(1):108-13.
150. Kalet AL, Gillespie CC, Schwartz MD, et al. New measures to establish the evidence base for medical education: identifying educationally sensitive patient outcomes. Acad Med. 2010 May;85(5):844-51.
151. American Association of Colleges of Nursing (AACN). Six AACN Member Schools Receive Funding to Support Efforts to Accelerate Health Research and Extend Precision Health. May 2019. Available at: https://www.aacnnursing.org/News-Information/Press-Releases/View/ArticleId/23877/all-of-us-funding
152. University of Michigan School of Public Health. Master of Science in Health Services Research. Available at: https://sph.umich.edu/hmp/programs/hsr.html
153. Mullins CD, Cooke CE, Cooke JL. Applications of Pharmacoeconomics for Managed Care Pharmacy. J Managed Care Pharm 1997; 3: 720-726
154. Husereau D, Drummond M, Petrou S, et al. ISPOR Health Economic Evaluation Publication Guidelines - CHEERS Good Reporting Practices Task Force. Consolidated Health Economic Evaluation Reporting Standards (CHEERS) — explanation and elaboration: a report of the ISPOR Health Economic Evaluation Publication Guidelines Good Reporting Practices Task Force. Value Health. 2013 Mar-Apr;16(2):231-50
155. Kaakeh R, Hutton DW, Funk K, et al. Cost-Effectiveness of 3 Statin Sample Policies in Post–Myocardial Infarction Patients. Am J Pharm Benefits. 2013;5(2):e36-e45
156. Danzon PM, Drummond MF, Towse A, et al. Objectives, Budgets, Thresholds, and Opportunity Costs- A Health Economics Approach: An ISPOR Special Task Force Report [4]. Value Health. 2018 Feb;21(2):140-145.
157. Patel TS, Kaakeh R, Nagel JL, et al. Cost Analysis of Implementing Matrix-Assisted Laser Desorption Ionization-Time of Flight Mass Spectrometry Plus Real-Time Antimicrobial Stewardship Intervention for Bloodstream Infections. J Clin Microbiol. 2017 Jan;55(1):60-67
158. Kaakeh R, Sweet BV, Reilly C, et al. Impact of drug shortages on U.S. health systems. Am J Health Syst Pharm. 2011 Oct 1;68(19):1811-9.
159. Neel ST. A cost-minimization analysis comparing immediate sequential cataract surgery and delayed sequential cataract surgery from the payer, patient, and societal perspectives in the United States. JAMA Ophthalmol. 2014 Nov;132(11):1282-8.
160. Davis GE, Schwartz SR, Veenstra DL, et al. Cost comparison of surgery vs organ preservation for laryngeal cancer. Arch Otolaryngol Head Neck Surg. 2005 Jan;131(1):21-6.
161. Men P, Yi Z, Li C, et al. Comparative efficacy and safety between amisulpride and olanzapine in schizophrenia treatment and a cost analysis in China: a systematic review, meta-analysis, and cost-minimization analysis. BMC Psychiatry. 2018 Sep 5;18(1):286.
162. Caro JJ, Ward A, Deniz HB, et al. Cost-benefit analysis of preventing sudden cardiac deaths with an implantable cardioverter defibrillator versus amiodarone. Value Health. 2007 Jan-Feb;10(1):13-22.
163. Najafzadeh M, Andersson K, Shrank WH, et al. Cost-effectiveness of novel regimens for the treatment of hepatitis C virus. Ann Intern Med. 2015 Mar 17;162(6):407-19.

References

164. Prabhu SS, Kaakeh R, Sugar A, et al. Comparative cost-effectiveness analysis of descemet stripping automated endothelial keratoplasty versus penetrating keratoplasty in the United States. Am J Ophthalmol. 2013 Jan;155(1):45-53.e1.
165. Kaakeh R, Hutton DW, Funk K, et al. Cost-Effectiveness of 3 Statin Sample Policies in Post–Myocardial Infarction Patients. Am J Pharm Benefits. 2013;5(2):e36-e45
166. Baumann M, Stargardt T, Frey S. Cost-Utility of Internet-Based Cognitive Behavioral Therapy in Unipolar Depression: A Markov Model Simulation. Appl Health Econ Health Policy. 2020 Feb 15.
167. Wateska AR, Nowalk MP, Lin CJ, et al. Cost-Effectiveness of Pneumococcal Vaccination Policies and Uptake Programs in US Older Populations. J Am Geriatr Soc. 2020 Feb 22.
168. Center for the Evaluation of Value and Risk in Health, Tufts Medical Center. Cost-Effectiveness Analysis (CEA) Registry. Available at: https://cevr.tuftsmedicalcenter.org/databases/cea-registry
169. Pella JE, Slade EP, Pikulski PJ, et al Pediatric Anxiety Disorders: A Cost of Illness Analysis. J Abnorm Child Psychol. 2020 Feb 20.
170. Moran PS, Wuytack F, Turner M, et al. Economic burden of maternal morbidity - A systematic review of cost-of-illness studies. PLoS One. 2020;15(1):e0227377.
171. Girotra T, Lekoubou A, Bishu KG, et a;. A contemporary and comprehensive analysis of the costs of stroke in the United States. J Neurol Sci. 2020 Mar 15;410:116643.
172. Reimer AP, Zafar A, Hustey FM, et al. Cost-Consequence Analysis of Mobile Stroke Units vs. Standard Prehospital Care and Transport. Front Neurol. 2019;10:1422.
173. McMullen S, Buckley B, Hall E 2nd, et al. Budget Impact Analysis of Prolonged Half-Life Recombinant FVIII Therapy for Hemophilia in the United States. Value Health. 2017 Jan;20(1):93-99.
174. Mauskopf J, Earnshaw SR, Brogan A, et al. Budget-impact analysis of healthcare intervention. 2017. ADIS.
175. Drummond MF, Daniel Mullins C. Improving the quality of papers published in pharmacoeconomics and outcomes research. Value Health. 2013 Mar-Apr;16(2):229-30
176. Paulden M, O'Mahony JF, McCabe C. Discounting the Recommendations of the Second Panel on Cost-Effectiveness in Health and Medicine. Pharmacoeconomics. 2017 Jan;35(1):5-13.
177. Eddy DM, Hollingworth W, Caro JJ, et al. Model Transparency and Validation: A Report of the ISPOR-SMDM Modeling Good Research Practices Task Force-7. ISPOR-SMDM Modeling Good Research Practices Task Force. Value Health. 2012. Sep-Oct;15(6):843-50
178. Professional Society for Health Economics and Outcomes Research (ISPOR). ISPOR Good Practices for Outcomes Research Index. Available at: http://www.ispor.org/workpaper/practices_index.asp accessed 12/22/2015.
179. Gold MR, Siegel JE, Russell LB, et al. Cost-Effectiveness in Health and Medicine. New York, NY: Oxford University Press, 1996.
180. National Pharmaceutical Council. Guiding Practices for Patient-Centered Value Assessment. Available at: https://www.npcnow.org/guidingpractices
181. Perfetto EM, Oehrlein EM, Boutin M, et al. Value to whom? The patient voice in the value discussion. Value Health 2017;20:286–91.
182. Deloitte-AdvaMed. A Framework for Comprehensive Assessment of Medical Technologies: Defining Value in the New Health Care Ecosystem. Washington, DC: Deloitte-AdvaMed, 2017.
183. Pharmaceutical Research and Manufacturers of America (PhRMA). Principles for value assessment frameworks. 2016. Available at: https://www.phrma.org/Codes-and-guidelines/Principles-for-Value-Assessment-Frameworks

184. Sorenson C, Lavezzari G, Daniel G, et al. Advancing value assessment in the United States: a multistakeholder perspective. Value Health 2017;20:299–307.
185. Professional Society for Health Economics and Outcomes Research (ISPOR). Available at: http://www.ispor.org
186. Professional Society for Health Economics and Outcomes Research (ISPOR). Available at: http://www.ispor.org
187. Weinstein MC, O'Brien B, Hornberger J, et al. Principles of good practice for decision analytic modeling in health-care evaluation: report of the ISPOR Task Force on Good Research Practices--Modeling Studies. Value Health. 2003 Jan-Feb;6(1):9-17.
188. Danzon PM, Towse A, Mulcahy AW. Setting cost-effectiveness thresholds as a means to achieve appropriate drug prices in rich and poor countries. Health Aff (Millwood). 2011 Aug;30(8):1529-38.
189. Glick HA, McElligott S, Pauly MV, et al. Comparative effectiveness and cost-effectiveness analyses frequently agree on value. Health Aff (Millwood). 2015 May;34(5):805-11.
190. Bertram MY, Jeremy A Lauer, De Joncheere K, et al. Cost–effectiveness thresholds: pros and cons. Bulletin of the World Health Organization Bulletin of the World Health Organization 2016;94:925-930.
191. Edejer T, Baltussen RM, Adam T, et al. Making Choices in Health: WHO Guide to Cost-Effectiveness Analysis. Geneva, Switzerland: World Health Organization, 2003
192. Willke RJ, Neumann PJ, Garrison LP Jr, et al. Review of Recent US Value Frameworks-A Health Economics Approach: An ISPOR Special Task Force Report [6]. Value Health. 2018 Feb;21(2):155-160.
193. Stahl JE. Modelling methods for pharmacoeconomics and health technology assessment: an overview and guide. Pharmacoeconomics. 2008;26(2):131-48.
194. Brennan A, Chick SE, Davies R. A taxonomy of model structures for economic evaluation of health technologies. Health Econ. 2006 Dec;15(12):1295-310
195. Heslin M, Babalola O, Ibrahim F, et al. A Comparison of Different Approaches for Costing Medication Use in an Economic Evaluation. Value Health. 2018 Feb;21(2):185-192.
196. Mansley EC, Carroll NV, Chen KS, et al. Good research practices for measuring drug costs in cost-effectiveness analyses: a managed care perspective: the ISPOR Drug Cost Task Force report--Part III. Value Health. 2010 Jan-Feb;13(1):14-7.
197. Barnett PG. An improved set of standards for finding cost for cost-effectiveness analysis. Med Care. 2009 Jul;47(7 Suppl 1):S82-8.
198. Sculpher M. Using economic evaluations to reduce the burden of asthma and chronic obstructive pulmonary disease. Pharmacoeconomics. 2001;19 Suppl 2:21-5
199. Sculpher M. Using economic evaluations to reduce the burden of asthma and chronic obstructive pulmonary disease. Pharmacoeconomics. 2001;19 Suppl 2:21-5
200. Doran CM. Critique of an economic evaluation using the Drummond checklist. Appl Health Econ Health Policy. 2010;8(6):357-9.
201. Chiou CF, Hay JW, Wallace JF, et al. Development and validation of a grading system for the quality of cost-effectiveness studies. Med Care. 2003 Jan;41(1):32-44.
202. Ofman JJ, Sullivan SD, Neumann PJ, et al. Examining the value and quality of health economic analyses: implications of utilizing the QHES. J Mang Care Pharm. 2003 Jan -Feb;9(1):53-61
203. Aparasu RR, Bentley JP. Principles of Research Design and Drug Literature Evaluation. 2015. Jones & Bartlett Learning, LLC and Ascend Learning Company.
204. Leucht S, Kissling W, Davis JM. How to read and understand and use systematic reviews and meta-analyses. Acta Psychiatr Scand. 2009 Jun;119(6):443-50.

References

205. Barza M, Trikalinos TA, Lau J. Statistical considerations in meta-analysis. Infect Dis Clin North Am. 2009 Jun;23(2):195-210
206. Coleman CI, Talati R, White CM. A clinician's perspective on rating the strength of evidence in a systematic review. Pharmacotherapy. 2009 Sep;29(9):1017-29
207. Jones JB, Blecker S, Shah NR. Meta-analysis 101: what you want to know in the era of comparative effectiveness. Am Health Drug Benefits. 2008 Apr;1(3):38-43.
208. Pocock SJ, Stone GW. The Primary Outcome Is Positive - Is That Good Enough? N Engl J Med. 2016 Sep 8;375(10):971-9.
209. Kimberlin CL, Winterstein AG. Validity and reliability of measurement instruments used in research. Am J Health Syst Pharm. 2008 Dec 1;65(23):2276-84.
210. Atkins D, Briss PA, Eccles M, et al. Systems for grading the quality of evidence and the strength of recommendations II: pilot study of a new system. BMC Health Serv Res. 2005 Mar 23;5(1):25.
211. Atkins D, Eccles M, Flottorp S, et al. Systems for grading the quality of evidence and the strength of recommendations I: critical appraisal of existing approaches The GRADE Working Group. BMC Health Serv Res. 2004 Dec 22;4(1):38.
212. Guyatt G, Gutterman D, Baumann MH, et al. Grading strength of recommendations and quality of evidence in clinical guidelines: report from an American college of chest physicians task force. Chest. 2006 Jan;129(1):174-81.
213. Calvert M, Blazeby J, Revicki D, et al. Reporting quality of life in clinical trials: a CONSORT extension. Lancet, 2011;378:1684–5.
214. U.S. Bureau of Labor Statistics. Consumer Price Index Inflation Calculator. Available at: http://www.bls.gov/data/inflation_calculator.htm

Index

A

action plan · **125, 126, 135, 157, 158**
"acceptable threshold" · **152**
"added benefit" skills · **117, 118**
adjusting for time · **181**
administrators · **32**
advisory board of experts · **111, 113**
allocation of resources · **11**
analytical model · **161**
assumptions · **182**

B

base-case · **167, 183**
    base-case population · **148**
    base-case estimates · **167, 179**
baseline estimates · **167**
Blocks of Pharmacoeconomics Canvas
    Block 1 – The Question and Objective · **140**
    Block 2 – Perspective · **141**
    Block 3 – Competing Alternatives · **144**
    Block 4 – Type of Analysis · **147**
    Block 5 – Patient Population · **148**
    Block 6 – Location · **150**
    Block 7 – Time Horizon · **151**
    Block 8 – Decision Rule or a "Acceptable Threshold" · **152**
    Block 9 – Design a Conceptual Framework · **157**
    Block 10 – Consequences Model Inputs: Appropriate Outcome Measures · **166, 168**
    Block 11 – Cost Model Inputs: Appropriate Costs · **170**
    Block 12 – Human Resources · **173**
    Block 13 – Sources of Data (Data Sources) · **174**
    Block 14 – Retrieval of Evidence · **176**
    Block 15 – Data Collection · **176, 179**
    Block 16: Adjusting for Time · **181**
    Block 17 – Assumptions · **182**
    Block 18 – Sensitivity Analysis · **182**
    Block 19 – Limitations · **185**
    Block 20 – Frame the Results · **186, 187**
    Block 21 – Frame the Discussion, Recommendation and Conclusion · **190**
    Block 22 – Full Evaluation and Recap · **191**
budget impact analysis · **79**

C

clinical decisions · **28**
clinical measures · **43**
clinical outcomes · **168**
collaborators · **111, 113**
collecting data · **178**
communication strategies · **82, 99, 102, 124**
Comparison Across Economic Analyses (Figure) · **63, 147**
Comparison of Competing Alternatives or Options (Table) · **146**
competing alternatives · **144**
conceptual framework · **157**
conduct team · **108**
conducting pharmacoeconomic analyses · **133, 156**
core skills · **117**
core team · **109**
cost · **18, 64, 166, 170, 172**
cost consequence analysis · **78**
cost inputs · **170**
cost of illness · **78**
cost-benefit · **63, 64, 67, 69, 147**
cost-benefit analysis · **67**
Cost-Benefit Analysis (Table) · **69**
cost-effectiveness · **57, 63**
cost-effectiveness analysis · **57, 63, 70**
Cost-Effectiveness Analysis (Table) · **74**
cost-effectiveness plane · **71**
cost-effectiveness threshold · **75, 153**
cost-minimization · **63, 64, 65, 66**
cost-minimization analysis · **65, 147**
Cost-Minimization Analysis (Table) · **66**
cost-per-QALY · **58, 75**
cost-utility · **63, 75**
cost-utility analysis · **63, 75**
Cost-Utility Analysis (Table) · **77**
creators · **84, 91, 92, 93**

D

data collection · **101, 117, 159, 179**
Data Collection for Each Model Input Estimates (Table) · **180**
Data Collection for Each Study for Comparison Across Studies (Table) · **180**
data sources · **173, 174**
decision analysis · **160, 161**
decision criteria · **31, 37, 58, 63, 65, 68, 69, 73, 74, 77, 154**
decision models · **161, 162**
decision questions · **30, 35**
decision rule · **75, 152**
decision tree · **161, 162, 163, 164**
decision-analytic models · **161**
decision-makers · **28, 32, 33, 35, 113**
decision-making · **28**
decision-making questionnaire · **34**
decision-making process · **35**
demonstrate value · **23**

Index

design meetings · **125**
designer mindset · **83**
design process · **83**
designer · **83, 84, 91, 92, 93**
deterministic sensitivity analyses · **183**
develop an action plan · **135, 158**
differences with value · **23**
direct medical costs · **44, 172**
direct non-medical costs · **172**
discounting · **181**
disease-specific instruments · **76**
doer · **91, 92, 93**
Does it make clinical sense? · **191, 192**
domains of The Process · **82, 97**
dominant · **70, 71, 189**
dominated · **70, 71, 189**
drug information specialist · **111, 113**

E

economic decisions · **29**
economic measures · **44**
effectiveness · **45**
efficacy · **45**
efficiency · **17**
elements that influence time · **47**
elements of The Process · **82, 99**
environment · **82, 97**
equity · **18**
experience · **19**
evaluate team · **108**
evaluating or interpreting a pharmacoeconomics analysis · **133**
evidence · **176**
Examples of Detailed Features of the Product or Service to Compare Across Competing Options (Table) · **146**

F

four pillars of the pharmacoeconomics base · **82, 88, 89**
Frame 1: Define the Criteria · **139**
Frame 2: Frame the Methods then Conduct and/or Evaluate · **156**
Frame 3: Evaluate the Output · **186**

G

generalizability · **59, 60**
generic instruments · **76**
global perspectives · **58**
goals · **15**
goal of the Pharmacoeconomics Canvas · **132**
guidance · **129**

H

health economics · **53**
health economist · **111, 112**
health outcomes · **17**
health states · **165**
Healthcare – Innovation – Outcomes (HIO) Triad · **39**
healthcare providers · **32, 111, 112**
how we learn pharmacoeconomics · **61**
human resources · **14, 173**
humanistic measures · **44**
humanistic outcomes · **168**

I

Incremental Cost-Effectiveness Ratio (ICER) · **70, 71, 154, 188, 189**
indirect costs · **172**
individuals · **82, 90, 91, 94**
Individuals (Figure) · **91**
industry leaders · **32**
inflation · **181**
information sources · **174**
innovation · **39**
intangible costs · **172**

L

lead designer · **124**
learn pharmacoeconomics · **61**
lifecycle of a pharmacoeconomics analysis · **86, 87**
Lifecycle of a Pharmacoeconomics Analysis (Figure) · **87**
limitations · **45, 59, 60, 164, 180, 185**
Literature Review Database (Table) · **149**
location · **150**

M

markov models · **161, 165**
medication formulary decisions · **29, 56**
mentors · **111, 116**
model cycle · **165**
model inputs · **166**
"must-haves" skills · **117**

N

needs assessment · **34**

O

objective · **139, 140**
opportunity costs · **144, 152**
outcomes · **40, 42**
outcome measures · **41, 168**
outcomes research · **41**
overview of economic analyses · **63, 64**
Overview of Economic Analyses (Table) · **64**

P

partners · **111, 113**
patients · **32**
patient advocates · **111, 115**
patient population · **148**
payers · **32**
pharmacoeconomics helpline · **109**
performing outcomes research · **42**
perspective · **118, 139, 141**
pharmacoeconomics · **53**
    pharmacoeconomics base · **82, 88**
    pharmacoeconomics canvas · **129, 137, 138, 193**
    pharmacoeconomics conduct team · **108**
    pharmacoeconomics evaluate team · **108**
pharmacy and therapeutics committee · **32**
pillars · **82, 88, 89**
policymakers · **32**
preferences · **153, 169**
presentation of the data · **188**
probabilities · **158, 161, 162, 164, 165**
probabilistic sensitivity analyses · **183, 184**
public health officials · **32**
publication to practice gap · **59, 60**

Q

quality · **17, 177**
quality-adjusted life years · **31, 57, 75**
question · **139, 140**

R

real-world data · **47**
real-world decision-making · **47, 48**
realities on the ground · **15**
recruiting team members · **121**
researchers · **83, 84, 112**
resources · **173, 174**
retrieval of evidence · **176**
reviewing outcomes research · **42**

S

satisfaction · **19**

scarcity · **11**
sensitivity analyses · **182, 189**
simple decision tree · **163, 164**
sources of data · **174**
standard guidelines · **129**
standardized form · **179**
starting point · **57**
statement on use of pharmacoeconomics canvas · **136**
"statement of intended use" · **130**
statistician · **111, 112**
study components · **82, 97, 98**
study designs · **159**
summary of base case results · **189**

T

tangible costs · **172**
team · **107**
team archetype · **111**
team assessments · **122**
Team Assessments Tracking System (Table) · **123**
team culture · **127**
team types · **108**
The Process · **82, 97, 99**
thresholds · **153**
time · **97, 98**
time horizon · **139, 151, 179**
transition probabilities · **158, 165**
transparency · **129, 135, 160, 185, 187**
type of analysis · **63, 139, 147**
types of costs · **171, 172**
Types of Costs (Table) · **172**

U

universal questions · **135**
user · **91, 92, 93**
utility · **169**

V

value · **21, 94**
value assessment frameworks · **25**
"value process" · **24**

W

What is driving the model? · **191, 192**
What went into the model? · **191**
Where and when can I use this information? · **191, 192**
willingness-to-pay · **68, 153**

Index

Tables

Overview of Economic Analyses · **64**
Cost-Minimization Analysis · **66**
Cost-Benefit Analysis · **69**
Cost-Effectiveness Analysis · **74**
Cost-Utility Analysis · **77**
Lifecycle, Design & Build, The Process (Domains, Elements) · **82**
Team Assessments Tracking System · **123**
Comparison of Competing Alternatives or Options · **146**
Examples of Detailed Features of the Product or Service to Compare Across Competing Options · **146**
Literature Review Database · **149**
Types of Costs · **172**
Data Collection for Each Study for Comparison Across Studies · **180**
Data Collection for Each Model Input Estimates · **180**

Figures

Cost-Effectiveness Plane · **71**
Lifecycle of a Pharmacoeconomics Analysis · **87**
Individuals · **91**
The Pharmacoeconomics Canvas · **137, 138, 193**
Frame 1: Define the Criteria · **139**
Comparison Across Economic Analyses · **63, 147**
Frame 2: Frame the methods then conduct and/or evaluate · **156**
Simple Decision Tree · **163**
Frame 3: Evaluate the Output · **186**

About the Author

Dr. Rola Kaakeh is the CEO of Salus Vitae Group and adjunct faculty at the Northwestern University Feinberg School of Medicine. She is a fellowship-trained licensed pharmacist with nearly 15 years of experience in academic, corporate, and pharmacy practice settings. Dr. Kaakeh advises a wide range of institutions, including universities, corporations, consultancies, professional associations, non-governmental and humanitarian organizations, and startups. Her areas of focus include national policies and institution-specific initiatives that address healthcare topics covering access, delivery, and outcomes. She has won numerous awards and presented on several global stages to address pressing healthcare issues. Dr. Kaakeh started university at the age of 10 as a gifted child, holds a doctorate in pharmacy from Purdue University, and completed a post-doctoral fellowship in pharmaceutical outcomes and health services research from the University of Michigan.

Empty Pages for Notes

Empty Pages for Notes

Empty Pages for Notes

Empty Pages for Notes

Empty Pages for Notes

Empty Pages for Notes

Empty Pages for Notes

Empty Pages for Notes

Empty Pages for Notes

Empty Pages for Notes

Empty Pages for Notes

Empty Pages for Notes

Empty Pages for Notes

Made in the USA
Columbia, SC
17 February 2022